Sitting Disease is Killing Us

Sitting Disease is Killing Us

Learn How To Prevent It

RUDY KACHMANN M.D.

Table of Contents

Preface · vii

Prisoner of the Chair · 1

Diet and Exercise · 4

Our Daily Calorie Burn · 8

Sitting Disease · 10

Total Daily Calorie Burn · 11

AOL · 12

LPL · 14

SUD · 15

Technology Caused the Problem, Technology Can Solve the Problem · · · · 16

Denial and Delusion · 19

The Master Disease of Our Time: Sugar Addiction · · · · · · · · · · · · 22

Fructose-Free for Two Weeks · 24

The Secrets · 25

Breaking Up the Body · 27

The Beginning of "Life in the Chair" · · · · · · · · · · · · · · · · · 30

Depression · 34

Music and Longevity · 35

The Dance of Life · 39

Great Immunity: "The Gold" · 41

Exercise · 48

Inflammation · 51

Sugar and Chronic Disease · 54

Sugar · 57
Early Diagnosis · 63
Motivation and Breathing · 67
Our Frontal Lobe Is in Charge and Motivates Us · · · · · · · · · · · · · · · · 72
Visualization · 77
You Can If You Think You Can · 82
Food Addiction and Plain Overeating · · · · · · · · · · · · · 85
Reversing Type 2 Diabetes · 91
Stress and Insulin · 96
The Brain and Eating: Rudy's Rules · · · · · · · · · · · · · · · 101
What's Your Situation: The Scoreboard · · · · · · · · · · · · 103
Ways of Eating · 104
What Does "Nutrient Dense" Mean? · · · · · · · · · · · · · · 105
Motivating Change · 108
Mind, Body, Spirit · 111
What Is Holistic Medicine? · 112
What's Going On in Your Life? · · · · · · · · · · · · · · · · · · 113
A Sense of Purpose · 115
Self-Discipline and Enthusiasm · · · · · · · · · · · · · · · · · · 119
Positive Thinking · 121
Don't Sit Still: Move · 125
I Was Blind, but Now I See · 128
Culture of Wellness Circle · 130
AOL: Activity of Living · 135
Children and Sitting Disease · 138
Summary · 141
About the Author · 143

Preface

We have an epidemic of overweight and obesity in the world. Unfortunately, it is causing the majority of our chronic diseases. This includes stroke, dementia, heart disease, and 60 percent of all cancers, autoimmune diseases, kidney disease, and many other illnesses. What is the cause? It's multifactorial. Factors include poor nutrition, lack of exercise, environmental factors, toxic chemicals put in food by the industry, fast food, and the high consumption of sugar products, including addiction to sugar.

Sitting too much is a big causative factor. It's been found that sitting for two to three hours is like smoking a pack of cigarettes. That has been scientifically proven. Dr. John Levine of the Mayo Clinic a number of years ago wrote a great book, *Move a Little, Lose a Lot*. I recommend you read it. The good news is that by following his concepts and my suggestions, we can turn this huge epidemic around, especially if you follow the recommendations I'm going to make, which are not that complex. You can achieve good health and wellness and avoid 80 to 90 percent of the chronic illnesses most people suffer from. I would recommend, among other things, not going on a diet but just eating different food. So the sacrifice is not calorie restriction. As a matter of fact, you might like this way of eating a lot better as the food is more delicious. It's achievable.

Dr. David Katz, the most experienced public health official in the country for over thirty-five years, wrote a famous book, *Disease-Proof*. He states that 93 percent of type 2 diabetes, 80 percent of vascular disease, and 60 percent of cancer can be avoided by controlling our fingers, forks, and feet. That is essentially what this book is all about. Frankly, it's great news that we can lead a healthy life if we follow some achievable recommendations. So read on, and let's participate in our healthcare.

Prisoner of the Chair

Being a "prisoner of the chair" is when you are not moving enough and are sitting too much. Some of us eat breakfast in bed (I did that for years), watch the morning news lying in bed or sitting in the kitchen, and then drive to work, sometimes for hours. Others drive for living. Just imagine truck drivers or delivery people. Almost all are overweight, although with some exceptions. Many restaurants and truck stops have awful food. I've been there. I spoke to the owner of about a thousand trucks; he stated 90 percent of his drivers are overweight. This is caused by lack of exercise, poor nutrition, and little availability of good food while on the road. According to federal law, truck drivers have to pass a new medical exam starting in 2016, I would say the majority of them are prediabetic and have not been properly tested. If they had a glucose-tolerance test, the majority would be out of work. It's scary that they're on the road, because blood sugar levels can change quickly. I know because I have treated a number of truck drivers, and frankly, they lack knowledge. They are good people, but screening for diabetes is incorrect most of the time. Proper health education could change all that quickly. It's the job of the federal and state governments, and they're not doing it properly.

I met a truck driver at Planet Fitness, a very nice gym. He weighed 360 pounds. I gave him a thirty-minute wellness talk, and when I saw him a few weeks ago, he weighed 210 pounds 1 year later, and his diabetes had gone away. Frankly, he looked like a movie star, and I did not recognize him. I even climbed in his truck to see what he was doing. He had a collection of nutrient-dense food, which he was eating on the road, and he had a small stove as well. For exercise he walked around the truck for one mile four times a day. It's just a plain good story.

The rest of us on average are sitting more because of our jobs. Some are lucky and move while they're working, as in some factory jobs, and even some office work involves a lot of physical activity. I stopped doing surgery two years ago, but the distance from my office to the hospital where I operated was almost a half a mile; besides, I stood all day while I was doing surgery. Let's face it; I got a good calorie burn walking, standing, and using my arms all day. I suspect my brain was also being exercised. Incidentally, I was a brain surgeon.

There are enzymatic changes in the endothelium of your blood vessels when you sit. It's the enzyme LPL, or lipoprotein lipase. It is located in the innermost layer of your blood vessels, and it is responsible for glucose and triglyceride metabolism. When you are sitting, its activity is reduced by about 50 percent. So you can see how easy it is to gain weight while sitting, when your metabolic activity has been cut in half. That's why sitting is like smoking.

The average person sits about five hours per day at work, then watches about five hours of TV at home. This has been very carefully studied. The average person takes about five thousand steps per day, the Amish farmer about eighteen thousand. That's a dramatic difference. No wonder we're sick. We shouldn't spend our time on the computer at work and at home, paying bills and sending e-mails, sitting down when using the phone, and playing video games for hours. I know some teenagers that do that till four or five o'clock in the morning. How many children do you see playing outside? Walking through my neighborhood for thirty minutes in the morning, I have rarely encountered children playing or adults walking. It's only me and the team of red-winged blackbirds following me that are getting some exercise. Just look around you in church or when you're waiting in a restaurant, and you will see what I'm concerned about. The combination of lack of exercise and poor food has a negative effect on our beltline.

If you're 5 to 10 percent overweight, you could be prediabetic. Many people with this problem have not been properly tested. A lot of the complications of type 2 diabetes occur in prediabetes, and 90 percent of prediabetics don't know they have it. I know because I do a lot of lunch-and-learns at corporations, and my vision is pretty good. I spend a lot of time trying to change that, but it's not easy. I do it in a lot of churches with the Daniel Plan.

The average American weighs about thirty-five pounds more than twenty years ago. It's worse in some racial and ethnic groups because of their history. African American slaves, for example, were starved and would eat sugarcane to stay alive. I actually saw some pictures of that in a book. This caused changes in their genetic structure, and now they become habituated or addicted to sugar more easily. This is not their fault, but they should be aware of it because we don't want anyone to have these horrible chronic illnesses. I see examples of this all the time. They spend a lot of time trying to change it.

The big increase in obesity has actually been in children and in the morbid obesity group, those above three hundred pounds. You can imagine the consequences if nothing is done about it.

Diet and Exercise

Reducing our food consumption, or starving ourselves, doesn't work, because it lowers our basal metabolic rate, or BMR, reducing calorie burn and delaying coming back up because our body thinks it's starving. That's based on evolution.

We are spending a fortune on gyms, but we're getting fatter. This is certainly not true of everyone. That's because we're not watching what we're eating, and we're sitting more, to the point where exercise becomes almost irrelevant. Actually, only about 3.5 percent of people exercise regularly. Researchers have found that around 20 percent of people say they exercise; they may sign up, but when the researchers track them, they find only about 5 percent actually follow through.

Fifty million claim they're working out, but don't. I checked this at Planet Fitness, a well-known and excellent gym. The person at the desk said perhaps only about 10 percent of their huge membership comes in on a regular basis. They tell their family, loved ones, and friends they belong to a gym, but the effect on their wellness is small because of their lack of participation.

Dr. John Levine from the Mayo Clinic thinks diet and exercise don't work, because they are not natural. The body thinks you're starving when you restrict calories, and it will come back to bite you. I agree with that. From reading the books of Dr. Joel Fuhrman and speaking to him personally, I'm completely convinced he believes that also. It's necessary to change the type of food that is eaten, essentially without restriction.

Frankly, we don't move enough. We are chained to the desk. We are addicted to sugar; it's the new slavery. We are a slave to refined carbohydrates, which are essentially sugar. Regular exercise, though, has great benefits. It improves our metabolism and decreases insulin resistance. It certainly does burn some calories, depending on the amount of exercise you're doing. The average person burns about 150 to 200 calories during one hour of exercise, but only 3.5% of the people do it regularly. Then again, it can be counted as part of your AOL, or activities of living. It also gives you the right mental attitude toward wellness. It's part of my AOL recommendations for wellness. Regular exercise reduces rates of cancer, produces neural plasticity, and encourages brain-cell growth and firms you up while you're losing some weight, and can cause muscles to grow, improve your balance, reduce falls, and give you a healthy appearance. Now that I'm semi-retired, I'm walking thirty minutes in the morning, working out one hour at Planet Fitness, playing about three hours of tennis a week, and constantly trying to increase my AOL, especially so that I can teach other people novel ways of improving their calorie burn during activities at home or work.

Working out regularly certainly would increase your calorie burn from all your AOL. Unfortunately, the literature indicates that only about 3.5 to 5 percent of people work out five days a week. Hopefully, that's not true. But then again, if your AOL burns calories slowly that is most convenient to you, maybe the critical need for that is not big in your life.

I work out in a gym for one hour a day; I spend about fifteen minutes on the treadmill, ten minutes on the elliptical, and ten minutes on the stationary bike. I do HIIT, high-intensity intermittent training. In this workout, you alternate between speeding up and slowing down, which improves the oxygen consumption of the heart and lungs. This can burn 150 to 200 calories an hour, depending on the intensity you are exercising at, of course. Then I do about thirty minutes of pyramid weight lifting, no more than twenty pounds. This way of exercising with intermittent training is better than running marathons.

Besides working at a desk, watching television is the biggest producer of sitting disease and its secondary health consequences. Working out during commercials, or just standing up or taking a little walk, helps prevent the sitting disease effect. Movement is the key. Just standing or walking is movement. A thirty- to sixty-minute workout three to five days a week is not enough. That is why AOL (activity of living) is critical. Use your imagination to pick some way at a work or home that is fun to use and inventive. Get your kids involved.

In summary, the easiest way to get back to health is by watching what you put on your fork, how you use your fingers, and how you use your feet. Eat the nutrient-dense way; increase your calorie burn, and then gradually increase your AOL, and you will make getting well much easier. Keep a diary at least for three to six months. It takes twenty-one days to establish a habit. Get your blood work done, check your weight, and make a plan. Failure means having no plan. Visualize your plan; it's a message to your subconscious mind.

The average individual sits almost ten hours a day. Increase your AOL (activity of living), the inventive and imaginative. It's about movement, not intensity. Try to do as much as you can at work; you are getting paid to be there, so figure out some AOL there. You and the company will profit from it. It's very important to track your activity. Don't live in delusion and denial.

Awareness is critical. If you're sick, act as soon as possible, and you'll recover quicker. Just a week in intensive care can cause tremendous muscle loss. Odds are you can do more than you think, or like the people around you may be thinking. Pressure them to help you. As a neurosurgeon, I saw a lot of patients getting better, pushed by the nurses to strengthen their bodies. Mild weight lifting and walking needed to be encouraged. Sometimes I would bring them light weights and work with them.

Move: you're worth it. Don't watch sports; play them. Reduce the time you spend watching other people play; you play instead. As we get older, we lose about three pounds of muscle mass a year; unfortunately, it's replaced by fat. When picking an exercise, pick one that is fun; you're more likely to do it. Whenever you're sitting, at home or perhaps an airplane, get up periodically and walk around. Walk at least thirty minutes a day. Play with the kids as much as you can; get them away from the television. Consider starting a garden; they can require a lot of muscle activity. Walk the dog twice a day, as I do. Both of us are of normal weight.

Take full advantage of every opportunity to exercise at work. A computer or work desk, which are just great, can have great value, consider demanding it. Park the car as far away from the office as possible and walk the extra distance. Stand up at least ten minutes every hour. Wiggle, jiggle, stand up, dance, and walk during lunch. Keep some light weights at your desk, and use them whenever you can.

Squeeze the wheel when you drive. If you are truck driver, try to stop three to four times a day and walk around the truck; figure out how many times around the truck equal one mile. Do it at every stop. I had one truck driver do that, and he went from 360 pounds to 210 pounds. He also learned to eat non-truck-stop food.

One study revealed that you burn 3.5 calories per minute when you stand up compared to sitting down, which burns 1 calorie. When you stand up, you burn 42 more calories per hour than when you're sitting. When you sit, you burn 2.6 calories per minute. Sitting less than three hours daily increases your lifespan. This has been scientifically proven. A study in Australia revealed that every hour spent in front of the TV increases the death rate by 18 percent. Sitting disease is the outcome of living a sedentary lifestyle.

Our Daily Calorie Burn

Our BMR (basic metabolic rate) is determined by our size, our weight, and the activity of our lungs, heart, brain, liver, etc. It's usually about 50 to 60 percent of our daily calorie burn. Based on your metabolic activity at rest. It's also based on our age and sex. It is difficult to change it. If you undergo major weight loss, because of the reduction in your size, your BMR will drop. This means it's harder to lose weight. If your body thinks you are starving yourself, it may take a long time for your BMR to get back up. Even if you're eating the same amount of food, you will find it more difficult to keep your weight down because of this reduction in your BMR. So about 50 percent of your daily calorie burn is difficult to change. Large people obviously have a bigger BMR because of their size.

Next, it would be good to know the amount of calories lost by the thermic effect of eating (TEF). For example, you would lose only about 4 percent of your calorie burn if you ate an all-fat diet. Ninety-six percent of those calories would be sitting on your abdomen or your buttocks within four hours. Very little would be converted to sugar and used up in immediate metabolic activity. So to keep track of the fat content of what you eat is critical.

If you were to eat an all-meat diet, you would lose about 20 percent of the calories through metabolism. That is certainly more than an all-fat diet but less than if you were also eating complex carbohydrates. Besides, it would be very bad for your kidneys and liver to metabolize that much protein. In addition, if the protein is from meat, it is usually accompanied by a lot of proinflammatory enzymes, which leads to increased rates of cancer and disease.

If you were to eat mainly vegetables and fruits, you would lose a tremendous amount of calories through metabolism of all that high-fiber food. First of all, vegetables generally are not calorie dense; second of all, they have a lot of fiber in them, which is difficult to digest. Besides, a significant amount of that will pass in the stool because of the fiber content. Generally, eating a high vegetable-and-fruit diet results in a loss of about 30 percent of calories through metabolism. When you add it up—it's not calorie dense to begin with, it has a lot of fiber, a lot of calories are lost in the stool, and 30 percent is lost through metabolic activity—just think of how many calories you're not taking in, because of this way of eating. You may lose 30–50 percent of the calories by eating this type of food. Just add it up; if you eat 2,000 to 3,000 calories a day, that's very significant. Remember, 3,500 calories equal one pound. If you're trying to lose weight, that makes it easy.

Then we have left an average of about 30 percent of your calorie burn based on your AOL. I like to include any regular exercise as part of your AOL (activity of living). The reason is that only 3.5 percent of people exercise regularly. If you read the work of Dr. John Levine for the Mayo Clinic, he calls this nonexercise activity thermogenesis, or NEAT. He puts regular exercise in a separate category. There's certainly nothing wrong with that, but I prefer to keep it in with your AOL, mainly because it's simpler. So I like to speak about AOL instead of NEAT. This is just my point of view. Both methods are trying to teach people about sitting disease, and that certainly is great. I think it's just a much simpler way of getting healthy.

So if we can increase our AOL and adopt a nutrient-dense way of eating, without dieting, it appears to me a reasonable way of becoming healthy, especially if you can do a lot of this AOL at work and increase the amount you're doing at home. In the following chapters, I will try to teach you to do that. I've had many patients become well and eliminate their type 2 diabetes and other chronic illnesses.

Sitting Disease

- Sitting two to three hours is like smoking one a half pack of cigarettes
- Work, TV, technology
- LPL enzyme turned off in capillary endothelium
- 50 percent reduction in glucose and triglyceride metabolism
- Lack of exercise
- Sedentary society
- Increase in overweight and obesity
- 150 million prediabetics
- 45 million diabetics
- Increased rates of cancer, heart disease, stroke, and so on
- Increased rate of aging and Dementia

Total Daily Calorie Burn

- 50 percent basal metabolic rate, or BMR
- Physiological activity of the heart, lungs, kidneys, brain, and so on at rest
- BMR—depends on age, sex, height, and weight
- Starvation reduces calorie burn and decreases BMR
- Thermic effect of food
  - Calorie burn of different foods
  - Lose only 4 percent of calories when eating only fat
  - Lose 35 percent of calories when metabolizing vegetables
  - Note that calorie loss can be large when eating fruits and vegetables
  - AOL – activity of living, 30-40%

AOL

- Calorie loss of your AOL (activity of living), including exercise
  - Walking the dog
  - Doing the dishes
  - Taking the stairs versus the elevator
  - Playing fun sports
  - Dancing
  - Standing while using the phone
  - Parking the car far away
  - Playing tennis, golf
  - Using computer desk
  - Lifting weights
  - Playing music
  - Watching ball games while standing
- Eating right
  - 70–80 percent highly nutrient-dense food
  - Minimal meat
  - Vitamins, minerals, and phytochemicals
  - Nutrient-dense food
  - Mosaic, rainbow, music, and orchestra of interaction
  - Eat nutrient-dense food of color
  - Vitamins, minerals and phytochemicals run the metabolic activity of your body and lead to good health, help with weight loss and fight diseases

Read

- *End of Dieting*, by Dr. Joel Fuhrman
- *End of Diabetes*, by Dr. Joel Fuhrman
- *The New Slavery – Sugar Addiction*, by Dr. Rudy Kachmann

Move

- Do exercise you enjoy
- Walk
- Dancing is the best exercise
- Yoga, tai chi
- Stand up – count them – about 50-100 daily
- Steps – count them – 10,000 daily

LPL

- Lipoprotein lipase, or LPL, causes sitting disease
- Located in the endothelium of the vasculature
- Eating a high-fat meal after sitting
  - Causes blood fats to increase 180 percent
  - Turns your blood serum dark
  - Can cause sudden death
- White and red muscle twitch fibers – slow and fast
- Vigorous exercise affects white fibers mainly
- AOL activity hits the red fibers mainly
- Prolonged sitting
  - Increases risk of heart attacks and strokes x3
  - Doubles the risk of metabolic syndrome
  - Shrinks muscles
  - Decreases balance and increases falls
  - Decreases longevity

SUD

- Use a stand-up desk at work (SUD)
- Computer treadmills are available now
- Use below desk devices for exercise
- $E=mc^2$—Einstein thought of it while riding a bike
- Child obesity—50 percent increase in ten years
- AOL increases brain growth, neuroplasticity
- Dancing is best exercise and Increases brain growth 76 percent
- Work activity
  - Invent AOL at work
  - Cheaper and easier
  - Use a stand-up desk
  - Keep an AOL (activity of living) diary

Technology Caused the Problem, Technology Can Solve the Problem

TV, phones, iPads, and computers are a part of the reason we sit a lot more. Certainly they're part of the obesity epidemic. Truck drivers sit all day. Many of them are prediabetic or diabetic because of increasing obesity and diabetes. Most people are driving instead of walking to work now. Some commute for hours, whether by car or on a train or a bus. One of my relatives uses all three and then sits at his desk for eight hours. You think he's got sitting disease? Your eyes could give me the answer.

Most of us are suffering from sitting disease today. If you're sitting more than one to three hours, the enzymatic structure in your cells, especially the inner layer of your blood vessels, called the endothelial cells, will reduce the activity of the enzyme LPL, which cuts fat and sugar metabolism about 50 percent. It's like smoking a pack or two of cigarettes. This has been scientifically proven. Sitting disease is the new smoking. We can start to turn things around by increasing our AOL, or what Dr. John Levine from the Mayo Clinic calls nonexercise activity thermogenesis, or NEAT.

There are a number of technical devices out now that could turn things around. The Mayo Clinic talks about using a device called the Gruve. I bought it and found it a bit difficult to use. A lot of people use a device called Fitbit and have found it useful. I know a family of four who use the Fitbit daily to encourage one young child in particular to move more. It's working. They told me about an incident the other day when the parents couldn't go to sleep because the child was running up and down the stairs, trying to get the Fitbit to ten thousand. Incidentally, my research indicates that we burn one calorie per twenty steps on average. Certainly it depends a bit on how the steps are taken, but that's the average. In other words, ten thousand steps burn on average about five hundred calories. It also makes you pay more attention to your health in general, including possibly what you eat.

Many devices are being used and coming to market and are very popular. The new smartphones have built-in pedometers. They also have many other apps and trackers that could be helpful. Plus there's a lot of information about tracking calories, tracking exercise, free recipes, and so on that can be of value. Many new apps tell you calories burned and amount of weight lost with the number of steps you are taking. Some even track the total vibrations of your body per day and then the calories burned.

I do think, though, that the exact amount of calories consumed or burned per day is difficult to calculate. The reason is it depends on your BMR, and that has to be calculated and related to the daily calorie burn. Then again, remember I'm giving you average figures.

Technology can help you become mindful of what you are doing and eating, how much you are exercising, and the amount of AOL you are doing. Clearly, the Fitbit is doing a lot for the child I'm speaking about, as well as his brother and parents.

Most people take 4,000–5,000 steps a day. An Amish farmer takes about 18,000 steps a day. The Mrs. about 14,000 steps a day. You can increase to 10,000 steps gradually, which is recommended instead of one big jump. Some do it, but it's not that easy. Setting a goal of increasing by 1,000 steps weekly is a good goal. A walk during lunch could provide about 2,000 steps. Maybe you could hit the treadmill or walk thirty to sixty minutes daily. The secret is to see whether you can increase it while you're working; it will make life a lot easier for you and give you more hours in the day, hopefully to do AOL at home and not to watch TV.

If you can afford it, try a fitness tracker on your iPhone or iPad. Some pedometers also track your heart rate and sleeping habits and pick up every vibration of your muscles and movement. They're a bit more expensive, but you might some find them very useful. Using this technique can be motivational and helpful.

Some people use a stand-up desk, or SUD, or a treadmill connected to a computer. You can burn about two hundred calories in one hour. Can you imagine, if you did that regularly, how much you would increase your AOL daily? If you also watch what you eat, weight loss could be simple. Remember, if you increase your AOL and burn two hundred more calories a day that amounts to a twenty-pound weight loss in one year. That's absolutely true and wonderful news. There also lots of other types of small exercise equipment you could use at your desk, including small things that increase foot movement, light weights, and so on. Your employer should pay for some this equipment; your employer will recoup the expenses easily in reduced healthcare costs. Work absence because of illness will steadily go down. Actually, many employees would be interested in this, if this were to become available in many offices.

Standing increases calorie burn x3, so standing at work burns calories. A standing desk can be simple or complex. Remember, when you're standing, you're not sitting, and you will be healthier. I highly recommended treadmills with computers. You could even use them at home, watching a movie or a ball game while standing up. Some treadmills are so small they can be folded under your desk or hidden at home if necessary. You can even get a walking treadmill with a desk, and they're just great.

Denial and Delusion

D r. Jeffrey S. Bland wrote a great book called *The Disease Delusion*, endorsed by the famous Dr. Mark Hyman. They are singing the same tune as I am and throw in some other great information. I highly recommend you read it. Dr. Mark Hyman has an excellent website, and I recommend you print off his *How to Speak to Your Doctor*, forty very informative pages. On page 11 he recommends the test you should get for good screening. To me those forty pages are the bible of prevention. I recommend you print off those forty pages and read them periodically. This will lead to disease prevention and a long life.

For one thing on page 11 do that testing and we are able to detect if you are on a path to type 2 diabetes and chronic disease or not. Prevention, stopping, and reversal are my game; become a player. You may need to turn the ship around and move into friendlier waters. Denying the potential storm won't help you. The earlier you become aware of your state of health, the easier it will be to get on the right road if that is necessary. Remember, the wrong road can lead to disability or early death. Yes, it does happen. Don't live in denial.

About 50 percent of Americans have at least one chronic disease; at age sixty, generally they have at least two. Fully 90 percent of these diseases are avoidable with good health habits. The CDC estimates that 78 percent of healthcare spending is on avoidable chronic illnesses. This is a healthcare problem all over the world. In Minnesota 95 percent of the people are prediabetic or diabetic.

DALY is the acronym for disability-adjusted life year. The DALY describes the years of life that we lose because of premature mortality and disability. This gives you a more realistic look at your life. Let's face it; if you have type 2 diabetes, your DALY may be ten to twenty years, if you live that long. It is mostly avoidable.

From 1990 to 2010, there was a great increase in our DALY. Heart attacks, strokes, metabolic disease, type 2 diabetes, dementia, and cancer turned into a global epidemic. We now have a "pill for the ill" to treat your problem, instead of "lets try wellness first" unless it's an emergency. We teach medical students around the world "crisis medicine." I recently reviewed the teaching methods done at Indiana University during my alumni meeting. A professor told us what they taught. They spend only two hours on teaching nutrition in four years. For Pete's sake, poor nutrition results in 90 percent of our chronic diseases. Wake up, medical schools. All doctors should know wellness in detail; I would estimate less than 5 percent do. There is a disconnect going on. The pharmaceutical industry pays for a lot of the research at medical schools, and maybe that's the origin of this "pill for the ill." It's not healthcare, its "sick care". Chronic illness is more than one-step or misstep in it, so wellness is not like an antibiotic, where one step may kill those bacteria. As I stated in my chapter, the "wheel of wellness" has many steps in it.

So we now have polypharmacy trying to hit the individual targets. Side effects are numerous and kill about a hundred thousand people a year. Just watch all the advertisements on TV and the description of the complications that could occur; it's frightful. Certainly, some medications are very helpful. In Europe they don't allow the pharmaceutical industry to advertise, or at least it's severely restricted. We are a nation of pills. In some countries it's even worse; in Japan, for example, it's frightening. Adverse drug reactions are common. Many are unreported because they killed the patient. I see many patients in the late stages of life on fifteen to twenty medications.

Many of us are aware of this, especially patients, but they don't know what to do about it. The healthcare providers, nurses and medical schools messed up. It's a little easier, though, just to practice "pill for the ill" and not bother to speak to the patient. Shameful.

Genetic inheritance is not our future most the time; it's what we do that is. I encourage you to watch my lecture on epigenetics at KachmannHealth. com. The good news is that over 90 percent of how you use your fingers, what put on your fork, and how you use your feet can determine your future. It's not the genes in what you heard most of the time, but what you do, your lifestyle. That's the good news. Dr. Dean Ornish pointed that out to us in his famous studies. He wrote about preventing, stopping, and reversing heart disease. He proved a significant amount of heart disease is reversible through proper lifestyle. Rarely do I have a patient tell me that his or her cardiologist told him or her to read the work of Dr. Dean Ornish. I've read many of his books.

To get back to reality, get blood testing yearly, starting at birth. The cost is insignificant compared to the problem. Read Mark Hyman's *How to Speak to Your Doctor*. His book *Blood Sugar Solutions* is also an excellent read. You need to know your biomarkers, body mass index, and your blood tests and review your lifestyle. Drugs are rarely the complete answer. With some exception, drugs rarely cure the problem. They're expensive, and many have serious side effects. Lifestyle changes can correct 70 to 90 percent of the medical problems that we have today. Drugs do not achieve that.

The Master Disease of Our Time: Sugar Addiction

The Greeks spoke about the mythological giant Antaeus, who became stronger whenever he touched his mother, the earth. He was conquered by Hercules when Hercules held him off the ground. Twenty-five hundred years later, we have been lifted off the earth by the modern industrial complex. We have been held captive by the power of the industrial complex and the government. It's a world of thousands of processed food items made in a plant, along with their accompanying hormones, pesticides, herbicides, and genetically altered food that is killing us.

Dr. Norman Cleve, who was the chief medical officer of a battleship in World War II, was the first to propose that taking off the germ and the bran resulted in a sugary product that caused most Western diseases. He set out the concept that most Western diseases were caused by consuming refined-carbohydrate foods. He felt the fundamental problem lay in the fact that Westerners had a profound change in their diet in a very short period of time, which did not allow for evolutionary adaptation. Dr. D. P. Burkett from England, also way ahead of his time, agreed with that. Dr. Robert Lustig also agrees.

The mass incrimination of sugar and white flour as the cause of a lot of Western diseases was first advanced by Dr. Cleve in 1956. Dr. Cleve used the term "the saccharine disease" and published his book by the same name in 1956, so I think we may need to give him the original credit for this concept. He also stressed the term "simplicity," reminding us that the biggest advances in humanity have been simple. He called saccharine a refined carbohydrate in that it caused a carbohydrate disease. No distinction between the twin's glucose and fructose, and especially the evil twin fructose, was made, because science had not advanced far enough. The metabolism of fructose was likely not known at that time. Let's face it; the chemical formula for glucose and fructose is the same. Fructose is just an isomer of glucose. There is another simple explanation: high-fructose corn syrup had not been invented yet either.

Dr. Cleve brought up Charles Darwin's law of adaptation. He stated that there hadn't been enough time in terms of evolution for our bodies to adapt to this onslaught of new processed food. Both Dr. Cleve and Dr. Yudkin thought that sugar was the cause of the majority of Western diseases. Dr. Cleve thought that removing fiber exposed the carbohydrates' endosperm, causing constipation, varicose veins, diverticulitis, cancer of the colon, dental disease, type 2 diabetes, obesity, vascular disease, heart attacks, and strokes. Dr. Cleve also spoke about change in our intestines, the five hundred different bacteria and viruses living there, about one trillion of them, and how their reaction to produce carbohydrates (sugar) can result in a significant amount of disease.

We know of Dr. Ancel Keys entering the picture in the 1950s and the studies he did in the Mediterranean area. He proposed that fat causes chronic Western diseases, and eventually Dr. Cleve and Dr. Yudkin were thrown under the bus for thirty years. But now we have defined fructose, and its metabolic effects on the liver, as a cause of Western diet–induced diseases. The real evil twin, fructose, has been discovered, and we now know what it looks like. It has the same chemical configuration as glucose, $C_6H_{12}O_6$, but the atoms are arranged differently.

Fructose-Free for Two Weeks

We need to reduce the number of fructose enzymes. We can't eliminate all fructose, because some vegetables and other foods contain a small amount, which is of no consequence to you. Remember, usually you can consume up to thirty-five grams of fructose a day and be very healthy. The trouble is we are consuming sixty-six grams a day.

There is no need to count calories. Included is a list of foods that you can eat in the first two-week period, and you will notice that they contain less than 1 gram of sugar in a standard serving. The majority of them have less than 0.5 grams of fructose sugar.

The Secrets

Following are several secrets to a healthy diet and lifestyle that will help you along the way:

- All carbohydrates are not alike. Starchy, complex carbohydrates quell hunger and turn up our internal furnace, burning calories as heat and energy. High sugar, high fat, and simple carbohydrates increase hunger, food addictions, and cravings.
- The same starchy carbohydrates that prevent disease and premature death can stop and even reverse disease.
- The resistant starch in complex carbohydrates absorbs fat and cholesterol, while providing few calories and the feeling of fullness.
- Refined carbohydrates reduce the "good" HDL cholesterol and increase insulin levels, triglycerides, blood pressure, and fat stores—proven culprits in the development of inflammation, obesity, and diabetes and vascular disease.
- Foods that promote weight loss are high in complex carbohydrates, which take more energy, calories, to break down—a faster metabolism burns excess body fat.
- Consumption of complex carbohydrates helps the brain produce higher levels of serotonin, which reduces your appetite and increases your feelings of well-being.

- Reducing saturated fat without reducing refined carbohydrates works against the goal to lose weight and prevent or reverse chronic disease.
- Saturated fats increase artery-clogging LDL cholesterol. The unsaturated fats in fish, flaxseeds, and plant-based oils reduce LDL cholesterol, inflammation, and plaque within blood vessels.
- Trans fats offer what the Mayo Clinic calls "a cholesterol double whammy" by raising "bad" LDL cholesterol and lowering "good" HDL cholesterol. The greater the percentage of trans fats in a food product, the higher the risk for heart attacks and strokes.
- Try to limit olive and other cooking oils while trying to lose weight, and then use them sparingly. Fish, ground flaxseeds, and walnuts offer the benefits of omega-3 fatty acids without all the fat of oil.
- Animal protein raises cholesterol while plant protein lowers it. Meat also raises it.
- To get the minimum amount of protein you need each day, balance your vegetables with legumes and some nuts.
- To lose weight faster, choose raw foods such as apples, carrots, bell peppers, and other raw foods and vegetables. Snacking on crunchy foods slows the rate of digestion and provides thousands of disease-fighting nutrients.
- It takes thirty to forty calories a day to maintain one pound of muscle. The more lean body mass you have, the faster your metabolism is, and the greater number of calories you burn at rest. Do some weight training every week.
- The same starchy carbohydrates that promote weight loss can prevent, stop, and even reverse disease.
- Eat a diet of foods containing vitamins, minerals, and phytochemicals; it is the rainbow, symphony, and mosaic of these foods that leads to good health.

Breaking Up the Body

The chair we are sitting in is breaking our body apart without us being aware of it. Many don't realize that sitting for hours on end affects the physiology of the body. It affects the basal metabolism, circulatory system, nervous system, basic enzymatic system, and digestive system. We actually have a sitting enzyme.

The human body has about 850 muscles. They are greatly affected when not actively moving. Hours, days, weeks, months, or years of sitting will cause atrophy, or shrinkage, of our muscles. Our tendons, which are attached to our muscles, become shorter and weaker if we don't use them. Our bones also become softer and smaller when not used on a daily basis, and sometimes it takes only a few hours.

The physiology of inactivity has been extensively researched. The latter has shown according to Dr. Mark Hamilton that the reasons for sitting disease have been revealed. A lot of the original research also was done by Dr. Joan Vernikos and her fellow researchers at NASA in the 1990s. A lot of it was weightlessness research on space travel. It revealed that space travel increases the aging process without question. We now believe that that is inactivity, and that increases or decreases depending on how we use or do not use our body and feet.

There are a number of factors that are affected by loss of activity. For one, electrical activity in your nervous system decreases if you are not moving. The reduction in metabolic and enzymatic activity resembles death. Interestingly enough, they found that is your heavenly cholesterol, HDL, decreases and your lousy cholesterol, LDL, increases. That has metabolic effect and cause vascular disease. It starts a fire in your body, a fire we many times don't see till it's too late. It is related to LPL.

Your BMR decreases when you are sitting a lot, and your calorie burn goes down and leads to weight gain. Dr. John Levine from the Mayo Clinic has found that you burn between 700 and 1,000 calories in a typical office job and 1,400 if you stand—a big difference. Remember, 3,500 calories make a pound. An average farmer burns about 2,300 calories a day. An Amish farmer takes about 18,000 steps a day. Generally, 20 steps burns about 1 calorie. As already mentioned, standing would increase your calorie burn significantly. Walking at a leisurely pace two hours a day, you could probably lose about forty pounds in a year, science as shown.

The typical office employee puts on about sixteen pounds within eight months if sitting full-time. Reducing moving time and increasing sitting will turn off your sugar and triglyceride metabolism about 50 percent and increase your chance of developing diabetes. One study found that decreasing from 10,000 steps to 1,500 steps per day could lead to insulin resistance. One recent study found that a single day of prolonged sitting could dramatically reduce insulin activity in healthy young adults. Frankly, this is a dramatic finding. In a study done in England, researchers found a 43 percent improvement in blood sugar levels when people stood up. So there is scientific proof.

Sitting has also been proven to cause inflammation of your vasculature, which can cause chronic diseases, including heart attacks, strokes, cancer, and so on.

When you sit, the muscles in your calves that pump the blood back to your heart are turned off. This can be complicated by deep vein thrombosis, a potentially fatal problem. It has been found that breaking up sitting with light exercise every twenty to sixty minutes reduces the levels of biomarkers associated with diabetes. If you walk for two minutes every twenty minutes, it has been found; you can reduce your risk of diabetes. Studies have been done that prove walking for one hour on a treadmill-improved people's ability to speak clearly and think better. Their memories improved. Incidentally, it takes about four hours of training to use a treadmill computer properly so it does not reduce your work efficiency.

The Beginning of "Life in the Chair"

The first chair ever invented is in a museum in London, England. I have not sat in it; perhaps one day I'll touch it. Everything is done faster in the last two hundred years except us. The information age, the cloud, is speeding across the world in nanoseconds. But we are slowing down more every year. Maybe our body size has something to do with it. Detailed statistics predict that our overweight population will double in ten to fifteen years with its fellow travelers, chronic disease.

In studies done in 1860 by Dr. Edward Smith, he concluded the average factory worker in England was moving a great deal less than the agricultural workers. It was the beginning of the industrial revolution. He realized the health implications.

In 1885 the combustion engine was invented, and walking began to decline. In 1895 about three cars were produced in the United States, four thousand by the turn of the century. When Henry Ford invented the Model T, car production accelerated tremendously. In 1930, about five million cars were produced in the United States.

The new breed of office workers started to develop back pain, shoulder pain, carpel tunnel syndrome, and joint pain. They even eventually started a workers' compensation system to help employees. New office furniture was invented, which did help some.

There were cities built around cars, such as Los Angeles, California. Dr. John Levine from the Mayo Clinic describes in great detail in his books his true-life stories of the traffic around LA. To him it looks like the city was built by the auto industry to increase business. In the 1950s, city dwellers started moving out to the suburbs, and the real driving revolution began. Isn't it incongruous that we slowed down but our food became "fast"?

The first computers appeared in the 1980s. Over the next decades, people became even more tied to their desks with the new technology. They were handcuffed to the Internet with their machines, slaves of the Internet and slaves to sugar—"the new slavery." Sitting disease and the new slavery are a devil's bargain!

Now came the next evil that shackled us to the desk—e-mails. We now have about a hundred laborsaving devices to use, which have decreased AOL. Many of them are used to give us more time before we go to work; then we drive for minutes, sometimes for hours. Then we sit at work, on average about six hours. Then most of us eat fast food for lunch. Although about 10 percent walk during the lunch hour. Then we drive home. If you're a woman or a man you are expected to have dinner ready, so stopping at a fast-food restaurant for take-out dinner is not uncommon. We live in a very-little-time society. The majority of those foods have sugar in them and lead us down the path to being overweight. There has not been enough time in evolutionary history for our bodies to accommodate our changing sedentary behavior and foods.

Dr. John Levine for the Mayo Clinic studied agricultural workers and city dwellers in Kingston, Jamaica. He did so because health workers were beginning to see significant chronic disease among office workers. He found the office workers were sitting about six hours a day; agricultural workers were off their feet about three hours a day and did about twice as much physical activity. Dr. T. Colin Campbell in *The China Study* the exact same thing. He studied many different cities in China and recorded the residents' exercise patterns and what they were eating. He was able to relate chronic disease to sedentary behavior and poor food choices.

Around 1890, 90 percent of our people were rural; now it's less than 25 percent.

There is discordance between what we are doing and what nature designed us for. Nature did not design our bodies to sit. Studies have revealed if you eat and then sit, you don't use up the evil twins—glucose and fructose—and because of increased insulin from sugar metabolism, you gain a lot of weight. Insulin is an anabolic hormone and leads to obesity, arthritis, dementia, and cancer. Our bodies are designed to allow us to be continuously active, especially after eating. Compare yourself to a farmer or factory worker after eating, and you'll see that we're sitting most the time. Their AOL will burn a lot of calories and sugar, and the rest of us just get overweight.

Our molecular mechanisms are built on the premise of the body moving most of the time, because in evolutionary history, that's what we had to do to catch or gather food. Our bodies are revolting against the onslaught of inactivity and eating high-sugar foods, which is against our evolutionary history. Studies have proved the point. Our blood sugars rise for two hours after eating. They literally spike in a peak. If you walk or do something physical, the peak currents to a flat curve. Insulin secretion is lower because you're using up the sugar. So the chair is the diabesity gene. It causes diabetes.

This situation was scientifically studied by the Cricket Brain Trust and by the Heart and Diabetic Institute in Australia, according to Dr. John Levine. Yes, they proved it scientifically. Another group in Australia sentenced the people to a chair and then studied their blood sugars. More sitting was directly related to elevated blood sugars. Intermittent movement improved blood sugars dramatically. They determined that sitting for two hours reduces life expectancy by twenty-two minutes. Like smoking.

Japanese scientists found the less you walk, the higher your cholesterol. Swedish scientists proved that sitting increases heart attack risk. That certainly is no surprise since that's related to diabetes. Another study from Australia of twenty-two thousand people found that people who sat more than two hours had a 40 percent increase in premature death. They even found increased rates of cancer—again, no surprise since it is related to type 2 diabetes.

Sitting is actually more dangerous than smoking; it is the new smoking, just like sugar is the new slavery.

Depression

Depression is easy to understand if we feel no purpose in life, we may sink into the chair. The chair is home to the depressed, who have little interest in AOL. The major distractions - TV, the ball game, CNN, Fox News. We need more sugar because it's a quick fix; it's our cocaine that makes us feel better quickly. Maybe a little alcohol too, which contains sugar.

A walk is as good as Prozac, many say. I have noticed that after a forty-five- to sixty-minute workout at Planet Fitness, I feel like dancing while going out to the car. A lot of times I sing at the end of the workout—"Forever Young." At age eighty, I actually feel that way.

Vacations can lead to increased activity because you have more time. Yet others just eat out two or three times a day, and when they get home, they've gained five to ten pounds. So you must keep track and watch what you're consuming. Certainly a pound or two is okay, but a major weight gain could be difficult to correct.

Music and Longevity

Our inner ears are the concert halls of our nervous system. To music fans there are eager audiences of billions of neurons. Music can transform us to a higher level of brain integration. There is different music for different people.

Music can change mood quickly. Music lessons can improve our cognition; our ability to think improves. Dancing to music improves our longevity. Exercising to music causes brain cells to grow.

When I have my typical stressed-out day, I deal with life and death all day long. You have a malignant brain tumor; you're going to be paralyzed for life; how long do I have to live, Doctor? These are issues I face almost daily. These discussions have a great effect on me. Those problems are here today, and they will be here still tomorrow. How do I deal with that? How does the patient deal with that? As soon as I get in my car to drive across town to go to another hospital or play my friend in tennis, I turn on music that I enjoy, loud. I picked the music, and you know what? Within seconds, I am transformed. My neurons are firing a different tune, and maybe I'm singing to the music. I am visualizing the individual instruments being played; sometimes I'm conducting the orchestra. A friend of mine was driving behind me one time and called me on the phone. He said, "What are you doing, waving those arms?" I said, "I'm conducting." One time I drove to the wrong town, listening to Pavarotti, when attending one of my neurosurgery clinics in Ohio. We all need these "pauses" in time. There's a reason they play music in the dental office.

It has been found that we learn better with music. The Mozart effect has been proven by scientific studies. Music makes us more intelligent. Our memory and learning ability improve with music, especially the music of Mozart. No one knows clearly why, and there is a lot of speculation as to the reason. Music and dancing can be traced in evolution. Even ancients danced and made music. Music is found in every culture. Extra pleasure and emotions can be found in music. Memories improve with emotions, and you're more likely to form long-term, explicit memories. Music improves our will to live.

I've provided DVDs of Andre Rieu to a lot of nursing homes. I call them Rudy's concerts. Ten to fifteen people sit around in wheelchairs, watching the DVDs. Their happiness, alertness, and memories improve for two or three days, according to the nurses. I always played them for my aging mother, and I know it lengthened her life and always put a smile on her face, and happiness leads to longevity. A Parkinson's disease patient may act almost normal as long as his or her favorite music is playing. Clearly, this is a dopamine response.

Ecstasy is immediate pleasure. Music can do that. Music is the most immediate of all the arts and can produce ecstasy for a person in seconds. I experienced it once, when listening to Carmen singing "Meine Lippen, sie kussen so heiss," by Lehár, with the Andre Rieu Orchestra.

Playing music—taking lessons—leads to stronger brain cells, increases our neurotransmitters, and gives us a longer life with a sound mind.

Sound affects the whole body. Music causes increased neurotransmitter activity in the nervous system, and the brain generates a flood of anticipation, which we use to make sense of melody, harmony, and rhythm. It takes us over. Music is beautiful; it imparts optimism in our soul and brings happiness. It heals us.

Music and art provide the mind with careful, ordered experience, not the chaos of a migraine. It's like a perfect sunrise. The world is too messy. Music brings coherence. Great beauty usually arises from greater complexity. We alter our view of the world, at least for a moment. Nietzsche said this can be transcending. It puts us in another world for a moment, escaping our very chaotic inner world.

There are a number of ways that music affects us. It has been proven that music can slow down and equalize brain waves. Music affects our heartbeat, pulse rate, and blood pressure. It slows our stress response; we destress. Music reduces some muscle tension and improves body movement and coordination. That's why a lot of people exercise with music in their ears. For three or four minutes, play music while you do some stretching exercises. It will improve your movements and allow them to flow naturally. Lie down and listen to a slower movement or a Mozart symphony or a string quartet to relax you. Music can increase your endorphin levels, your own feel-good hormones. Music will strengthen your memory and learning.

When we are doing our everyday activities, we use the beta waves of the brain. When relaxing, we are using our theta waves. When we are sleeping, we have delta-wave activity. Yoga, meditation, and music decrease the brain-wave pattern and bring on theta-wave activity, a more relaxing mode. We live longer if we control our stress. Playing music can balance our intellectual brain and increase productivity and creativity.

It has been proven that music can improve your immunity and help prevent cancer and infection. Fifty percent of mothers giving birth did not need anesthesia when listening to music. They studied the music of Mozart, Beethoven, the Beatles, and Bach, and Mozart was a winner in the learning process. They're not sure why, but his music improved spatial perception, learning, and memory. Perhaps the rhythm, melody, and increased frequency of Mozart's music influenced the creative and learning regions of the brain. Mozart's music has creative and healing power. Mozart listened to his father's music while still in his mother's womb. Mozart said everything has been composed but not yet written down. What an imagination.

Bring music into your life. Listen, dance, sing, write, and promote it. Use CDs and DVDs and take dance and singing lessons. How powerful is your song? Mozart's music affects the electrical activity of the brain, according to the Royal Society of Medicine in London. It affects the hormones, neurotransmitters, and neuropeptides, the communicators of the human brain.

This is the day that the Lord has made; let us rejoice and be glad in it.—Psalm 118: 24

The Dance of Life

All types of dance are great. I'm speaking about the use of rhythm and movement to improve your longevity and intelligence. You have to use your mind to dance correctly. Ballroom dancing improves the mind and the body. Join a class, and do this one or two days a week regularly.

So whenever you are moving in rhythm, whether or not music is playing, you can consider yourself to be dancing. The dances of walking, jogging, biking, swimming, hiking, and even golf or tennis are following a rhythm. Keeping in rhythm means the timing of the swing, shot after shot, so you develop consistency. I play a lot of tennis. I have all my life, and really it's a form of dancing.

The effect of exercise on the immune system has been scientifically proven. Scientists have found that exercise has a direct effect on our white blood cells, the main cells affecting our immunity. After a few months of exercise, the levels of immunity-activating cytokines produced by white cells drop over 50 percent, while the levels of immunity-protecting cytokines rise about 35 percent, scientific studies have proven. Exercise is probably the single most effective way to lower inflammatory factors in the blood that cause cancer and vascular disease.

When physical activity is done through rhythm, it can be considered dance, a powerful way to get the most benefit from your exercise program. Pilates, for example, is an excellent way, as well as all other basic yoga activities. Qigong, tai chi, kundalini yoga, and dancing have the greatest effect on the inflammatory factors in your blood, the CRP (C-reactive protein) levels. Researchers have found greatly beneficial effects on anxiety and depression in people who performed exercises such as jogging, swimming, cycling, and walking. And music in rehabilitation and physical therapy programs for Parkinson's disease patients also have been shown to improve outcomes, when compared to standard physical exercises. Any rhythm to movement certainly increases the level of enjoyment and involvement in exercise classes. The addition of pumping rhythmic music to aerobic exercise classes encourages participation and increases satisfaction levels. Ask me and I will tell you—I own a yoga studio, and it works for our clients and us. Turning a standard exercise routine into a dance is more fun and less boring, and ensures that exercise is kept at their activity level.

Why does rhythmic exercise work so much better? Rhythmic contraction, alternating between flexion and extension, provides balance and strengthens both flexors and extensors equally. The nerve impulses that regulate muscle groups originate from signals in the brain and are transmitted along the spinal cord. With make movement rates of pattern in the brain and spinal cord that is also transmitted to our immune system. The same neurotransmitter chemicals released by the brain and nerve endings are sensed by our immune system. When a brain is dancing, so is the immune system. Human life itself consists of rhythms; it's quite possible that the immune system responds to these rhythms.

Who gave himself for our sins to deliver us from the present evil age, according to the will of our God and Father.—Galatians 1:4

Great Immunity: "The Gold"

The army, navy, air force, and marines (the immune system) that defend our health will determine our lifespan. Dr. Joel Fuhrman wrote another great book, *Super Immunity*, which was recently published, and it really is the gold of longevity and health teaching. I read a prepublished copy twice, and the publisher asked me to write a few words about it. I think that unless you fall out of an airplane, if you follow what is recommended, including the recipes in the back of the book, you have a 90 percent chance of living to be one hundred or better with a sound mind. It is all about a nutrient-dense way of eating, in which you eat the right macro- and micronutrients, vitamins, and minerals, the right complex carbohydrates, 100 percent whole grains, proteins, fats, and phytochemicals. That creates a strong immune system, a system that prevents vascular disease, heart attacks, strokes, cancer, infections, autoimmune disease, and so on.

The China Study, by Dr. T. Colin Campbell, proved that certain foods could provide health-promotion and disease-protection benefits. The study was done a few decades ago, but a lot of this information has been known for thousands of years. Natural plants are complex packages of biologically active compounds. The term "phytochemicals," which means "of-plant chemicals," represents the thousands of plant-source compounds that have profound effects on human health and immunity. Scientific discoveries have proven that the phytochemicals run the machinery of metabolism; they are the coenzymes that run the chemical reactions of our body. Our food, in other words, helps determine our resistance to disease and increases our longevity. The benefits of good eating habits have been largely ignored by 80 percent of the American people, resulting in a lot of diseases, poor health, and tremendous cost. Koreans, Japanese, Micronesians, South Americans, and Africans are being devastated by the sad, mad, toxic diet of fat, salt, and sugar. The human body can take advantage of the complex biochemical compounds found in plants that we can use to keep a normal weight, prevent illness, and heal previously damaged cells. We have stopped our overemphasis on vitamins and minerals and started paying attention to the defense and repair mechanism of our body's twenty-five thousand phytochemicals. The phytochemicals are bioactive, plant-derived chemical compounds important for the growth and survival of the planet. Plants use these phytochemicals to defend themselves against their enemies—funguses, viruses, bacteria, and animals. The human immune system evolved to be dependent on phytochemicals for its optimal functioning.

Superior nutrition is the secret of the "superior immunity" that Dr. Joel Fuhrman writes about. You don't have to be a genius to realize that. There is great synergism of the human immune system and the phytochemicals of our plants. Animals and plants have developed a fragile, interconnected, and symbiotic relationship on earth. Now human beings rely on plants for health and survival.

We are what we eat. We are made from what we eat. Fat, salt, and sugar are not going to do it for you. That's what Americans eat 80 percent of the time, and look at our obesity rate—65 percent. One-third of our children are overweight. When we cultivate nutritional deficiencies in our body over long periods of time, especially in our formative years, it creates a lot of cellular damage, resulting in serious illnesses late in life. Advancements in nutritional sciences have created an opportunity for great health and longevity, preventing disease, including cancer, heart attacks, and strokes, which are well known in vegetarian societies. The chemical compounds found in vegetables, beans, berries, and fruits, when combined with nuts, seeds, mushrooms, and onions, fuel the miraculous self-healing and self-protective properties already built into the human genome. The American diet is a disaster of processed foods and animal products, which represent 85 percent of a mad, sad diet and are very low in nutrients, natural vegetables, and phytochemicals, and as a result of marketing are dramatically deficient in plant-derived, disease-fighting chemicals. We consume less than 10 percent of our foods as unrefined foods. Ninety percent of our food has been stripped of healthy fiber. We are not eating enough fruits, beans, seeds, or vegetables. We are missing the beneficial antioxidants and phytochemicals that repair the body and prevent disease. The carotene family—alpha and beta, lutein, zeaxanthin, lycopene, flavonoids, alpha-lipoic acid, quercetin, anthocyanins, lignans, pectin's, and so on—are among the great chemicals that can heal us and prevent cancer and numerous inflammatory diseases, and they are found in the vegetables and beans we eat. Since neither processed foods nor animal products contain a significant load of antioxidant nutrients and phytochemicals, the modern diet is dramatically disease prone.

Antioxidants are vitamins, minerals, and phytochemicals that aid the body in removing free radicals, which cause diseases that kill us. The vast majority of antioxidants are available to the body through fruits, vegetables, and other natural plants. Oxidative damage occurs when free-radical activity in the body increases and free radicals burst out of their cellular compartments to affect broader regions of the cells. Vegetables are so rich in antioxidant chemical compounds that eating a vegetarian, vegan, or nutritarian diet is an easy way to increase antioxidant capacity. Foods with great amounts of phytochemicals are cabbage, red peppers, carrots, green peppers, tomatoes, onions, broccoli, peas, squash, and mushrooms. A phytochemical-deficient diet is responsible for a weak immune system, resulting in disease and death at a young age. Populations with much higher amounts of vegetables in their diet have 50 to 70 percent lower rates of cancer and inflammatory diseases. The longest-living populations throughout history are the ones with a high intake of vegetables in their diet. Dr. Joel Fuhrman says that the phytochemicals are the most important discovery in human nutrition over the last fifty years. The concentration of phytochemicals is often highlighted by vibrant colors of black, blue, red, green, and orange—except maybe for the very healthy mushrooms.

The benefits of phytochemicals are as follows:

- Detoxifying enzymes
- Controlling the production of free radicals
- Deactivation and detoxification of cancer-producing agents
- Protecting cell structure from damage by toxins
- Fueling mechanisms to repair damaged DNA
- Introducing beneficial antifungal, antibacterial, and antiviral effects
- Inhibiting the function of damaged or genetically altered DNA
- Improving immune cells function
- Producing great disease-fighting antibodies, preventing cancer

The War on Cancer

Our cancer rates exploded between 1935 and 2005. The rate increased every year for seventy years. We've had an explosion of immune system–dependent diseases, allergies, autoimmune disease, and cancer.

Cruciferous vegetables are great anticancer agents. Green vegetables such as kale, cabbage, broccoli, cauliflower, and turnips are called cruciferous vegetables because as a flower, they have four petals like a cross. Cruciferous vegetables have a unique chemical composition. They make a sulfur-containing compound, where the cells are programmed to release ITCs, an array of compounds with proven powerful immune-boosting effects on anticancer activity. Eating cruciferous vegetables, chewing them and breaking the cellular structure, decreases cancer rates dramatically. Consuming mushrooms regularly is associated with a significant decrease in the risk of breast cancer. Frequent consumption of mushrooms can decrease the incidence of breast cancer 60 to 70 percent. So what's the solution? Dr. Fuhrman has a great formula: H=N/C. Health expectancy equals nutrient density divided by calories. There is our destiny.

To slow the aging process, we need to eat a nutrient-dense diet—vegetables, beans, and fruits, essentially all you can eat. Counting calories or portion control is not needed if you eat nutrient-dense foods.

Dr. Fuhrman's diet in his book *Eat to Live* has these features:

- Vegetable based
- Lots of fruits, beans
- Seeds and nuts
- Oil used sparingly
- Animal products zero to three times a week

The Standard American Diet:

- Grain based
- Lots of dairy and meat
- Lots of oil
- Major animal products
- Animal products five to seven times a week
- Focus on nutrient-poor calories

The Gold

Resistant starches are starches with a lot of fiber. The starchy foods will not be entirely absorbed because of their high fiber content. At least 30 to 40 percent of calories are lost in metabolism. They never enter the bloodstream. By contrast, the starch from a baked potato will have a high absorption rate because of lack of fiber. Calories in and calories out—the original concept was incorrect. Beans promote a sensation of fullness. They improve insulin sensitivity, decreasing diabetes. Beans promote good bacteria once the bowel has adjusted. Beans also have in them a lot of good essential fatty acids, which you need. The carbohydrates in them have a lot of fiber and will not all be absorbed, and you can eat a lot of beans because of that.

- Black beans—63 percent fiber
- Red kidney beans—56 percent fiber
- Navy beans—52 percent fiber
- Lentils—47 percent fiber
- Split peas—38 percent fiber
- Corn—32 percent fiber

A highly nutritionally dense diet will enhance cellular repair mechanisms and reverse disease. That is why this way of eating, which Dr. Dean Ornish recommends for preventing, stopping, and reversing heart disease, works. He essentially teaches the same thing that Dr. Fuhrman and I teach. This way of eating reduces the inflammatory response, suppresses genetic alterations, decreases free-radical activity, slows the metabolic rate, enhances DNA repair, and removes toxins.

What Is a Nutritarian?

A nutritarian is a person whose food choices are influenced by nutritional quality. It is a person who strives for more micronutrients per calorie in the diet and who recognizes that food is a powerful disease fighter with an effective and therapeutic effect. Nuts and seeds are good for weight loss. They have a lot of fiber in them, and they carry a lot of good essential fatty acids. You should eat at least one ounce a day. A lot of people get away with two ounces because they tremendously decrease the appetite.

How do you prevent, stop, and reverse vascular disease and diabetes?

- Eat at least fifty grams of fiber daily.
- Eat a 20 percent fat diet—fat from seeds, nuts, and vegetables.
- Eat sufficient omega-3—your essential fatty acids.
- Eat a high-phytochemical and high-antioxidant diet.
- Eat low-glycemic-index foods.

- Eat low-calorie, nutrient-dense foods.
- Limit animal products to two to three servings a week.

IGF

High levels of the hormone IGF reduce longevity and lead to cancer. Low levels lead to increased lifespan and decrease inflammation, decrease oxidative damage, increase insulin sensitivity, and slow the aging process. The amount of meat we eat determines our IGF level.

We have at least twenty major recommendations to live to be one hundred and be of sound mind. But what to eat by far will have the greatest effect. Your food selection is critical to your longevity.

EXERCISE

Learn to dance—one of the secrets of motivating yourself to wellness. All types of dance are great. I'm speaking about the use of rhythm and movement to improve your longevity and intelligence. You have to use your mind to dance correctly. Ballroom dancing improves the mind and the body. Join a class, and do this one or two days a week regularly.

So whenever you are moving in rhythm, whether or not music is playing, you can consider yourself to be dancing. The dances of walking, jogging, biking, swimming, hiking, and even golf or tennis are following a rhythm. Keeping in rhythm means the timing of the swing, shot after shot, so you develop consistency. I play a lot of tennis. I have all my life, and really it's a form of dancing.

The effect of exercise on the immune system has been scientifically proven. Scientists have found that exercise has a direct effect on our white blood cells, the main cells affecting our immunity. After a few months of exercise, the levels of immune-activating nasty cytokines produced by white cells drop over 50 percent, while the levels of immune-protective good cytokines rise about 35 percent, scientific studies have proven. Exercise is probably the single most effective way to lower inflammatory factors in the blood that cause cancer and vascular disease.

When physical activity is done through rhythm, it can be considered dance, a powerful way to get the most benefit from your exercise program. Pilates, for example, is an excellent way, as well as all other basic yoga activities. Qigong, tai chi, kundalini yoga, and dancing have the greatest effect on the inflammatory factors in your blood, the CRP (C-reactive protein) levels. Researchers have found greatly beneficial effects on anxiety and depression in people who performed exercises such as jogging, swimming, cycling, and walking. And music rehabilitation and physical therapy programs for Parkinson's disease patients also have been shown to improve outcomes when compared to standard physical exercises. Any rhythm to movement certainly increases the level of enjoyment and involvement in exercise classes. The addition of pumping rhythmic music to aerobic exercise classes encourages participation and increases satisfaction levels. Ask me, and I will tell you—I own a wellness studio, and it works for our clients and me. Turning a standard exercise routine into a dance is more fun and less boring, and ensures that exercise is kept at their activity level.

Why does rhythmic exercise work so much better? Rhythmic contraction, alternating between flexion and extension, provides balance and strengthens both flexors and extensors equally. The nerve impulses that regulate muscle groups originate from signals in the brain and are transmitted along the spinal cord. The same neurotransmitter chemicals released by our brain and nerve endings are sensed by our immune system. When our brain is dancing, so is our immune system. Human life itself consists of rhythms; it's quite possible that the immune system responds to these rhythms.

Rhythm is an integral part of life and is as old as history. Look at the old religions, tribal dancing, Hinduism. Dancing is thought to be the Arum of the universe. In Hinduism, you've probably heard of the ancient cosmic dance of Shiva. The frequency and randomness of all such sounds are considered to hold healing powers, as is the vocalization "ohm." Apollo, the son of Zeus and the god of medicine, was known as a dancer. In Sparta, authorities required parents to instruct their children in the art of dancing beginning at the age of five. Dancing is thought to be good for the body and overall health, as well as for the soul. In modern science, researchers have shown that music in rhythm produces measurable healing effects. Music has been proven to reduce stress and anxiety, as evidenced by multiple studies of heart patients who underwent catheterization and other unpleasant procedures. These patients' anxiety levels were significantly reduced when music was played during cardiac catheterization.

The brain uses a rhythm to heal. It is important to breathe in rhythm because it affects our immunity. Healers across many different cultures have employed dance to induce a trance as part of a healing ritual. The Chinese discipline known as tai chi, which originated more than eight centuries ago, is still used as a healing art. Tai chi creates a meditative state that is set to restore natural rhythms and balance in the mind and the body. When you combine movement with rhythm, you enjoy the double benefit of exercise and the meditative state; you lower the inflammatory factors in the blood. It is better when you have a bit of low-back pain to do some rhythmic movement. It's better than lying in bed or on the couch all day.

What action should you take?

- Walking for thirty minutes every day, in rhythm
- Swimming
- Doing entry-level aerobics and advancing over time
- Ballroom dancing—I did it for two years with two Russian dancers
- Biking
- Rowing
- Jogging
- Jumping rope
- Tap, hip-hop, square dancing
- Participating in competitive sports
- Practicing martial arts
- Getting a personal trainer
- Starting a weight-training program

INFLAMMATION

Our health is being destroyed by the effects of out-of-control inflammation. It's because of the toxic food we're eating and drinking. The epidemic of inflammation is a bigger cause of disease than our genetic structure is. The government is putting the majority of research money into gene research. But it's what we are eating and drinking that causes majority of our illnesses, yet we are devoting very few healthcare dollars to study that.

Being overweight and having metabolic syndrome and type 2 diabetes is the consequence of increasing insulin resistance in the blood. The causes of type 2 diabetes, which is all around us, are inflammation and insulin resistance. Inflammation is the monkey on our back, and the predecessor of insulin resistance. If there were no inflammation, we wouldn't have insulin resistance, or the resultant diseases and illnesses brought on by that. Dr. Mehmet Oz says, "Inflammation is the rusting of your arteries." Inflammation is a fire where you can't see the flames. It remains hidden for many years until you run some tests, and then it might be too late.

The immune system involves your thymus, spleen, bone marrow, and white blood cells—they are your army, navy, air force and marines, which are supposed to win the war and bring you back to good health. This happens when you may have a local infection. But in your body, it's an unending war, with your arteries and nerves involved with chronic infection because we continue to supply the body with toxic foods such as salt and sugar. As Dr. Herbert Benson from Harvard would say, there is a doctor living within everyone's body: the immune system, which knows how to repair things. We are attempting to repair the chronic inflammation but are causing a lot of damage in the process.

Your low-density lipoprotein, or LDL, infiltrates the interior walls of your arteries and capillaries; the inflammatory process jumps in with its macrophages to try to repair the problem and causes plaque formation instead. (Macrophages are powerful immune cells that are sent into the arterial walls and can cause thrombosis and in turn a heart attack.) This causes arterial narrowing and can lead to trouble. The inflammatory process occurs throughout the body, and in the brain it can lead to dementia. Eventually, inflammation leads to vascular disease, strokes, heart attacks, glaucoma, arthritis, kidney disease, neuropathy, and so on, and it can inflame your three hundred thousand miles of capillary blood vessels. The fact that the immune system plays a role in the onset of most major diseases has now been well proven. The immune system is a major killer stimulated by what we eat and what we do.

One million teenagers have metabolic syndrome based on inflammation. This bodes poorly for the future. Inflammation destroys the body by friendly fire. We are destroying our bodies by what we do or don't do. We're shooting ourselves in the head on a daily basis. Just look around you: most people are totally unaware of what they are doing to themselves, or they're just closing their eyes.

Our nation is dying from bad food. Oxidation is the process of aging. It's like trying new food with a decaying fruit like a banana. It makes your apple brown and its skin wrinkle. This is the aging process. Smoking is a cause of inflammation, and we all know that smokers may look twenty years older than they really are.

Anything that causes inflammation will in turn cause insulin resistance, and anything that causes insulin resistance will cause inflammation. They are the evil twins. We can easily identify inflammation from a sore throat, which is obvious, but the inflammation in our body can be hidden and turn into diseases and illnesses, resulting in chronic disease, disability, and death. The inflammation that drives obesity and chronic disease is invisible and doesn't hurt. It's a hidden, smoldering fire created by your immune system, which is trying to fight off bad food and sugar, fat, and salt in processed food, as well as smoking.

What triggers the inflammatory process? Sugar is number one, followed by refined carbohydrates, trans fats, and too many omega-6s from meat and from plant oils. Other triggers are artificial sweeteners, high-fructose corn syrup, food sensitivities, gut bacteria, genetic makeup, food additives and chemicals, factory-farmed meat, farmed fish, and gluten.

Mounting evidence underscores the critical role that inflammation plays in the development of type 2 diabetes. Dietary sugars and refined flours are the biggest triggers of inflammation. They cause insulin levels to spike and start a cascade of biochemical reactions that turn on our genes' chronic inflammation. Lack of fiber, too many inflammatory omega-6s, and not enough omega-3s, plus anti-inflammatory essential fats, lead to the development of systemic inflammation throughout the body. Food sensitivities and allergies also add to the problem. Many people have gluten sensitivity and not a true allergy. They get sick anyhow with many systemic-type symptoms, but it is not as deadly, unless they have celiac disease.

Many of the reactions and allergies are from a "leaky gut" created by proteins, by-products of food digestion that leak through holes in the gut. This occurs much more commonly with the reaction to genetically modified new foods, which have no evolutionary history. Many foods have been genetically modified. Our bread is not what it used to be; it's more of a Franken food, a product of industrial agriculture.

Sugar and Chronic Disease

How do sugar and carbohydrates cause chronic diseases such as heart disease, strokes, diabetes, cancer, and autoimmune diseases?

The mid-1800s started seeing the Western diseases of hypertension, osteoarthritis, gallbladder disease, and diabetes. Everyone seemed to get better when sugar was replaced by fat. Mind you, we're talking about the 1950s. So we've known for a long time that sugar and carbohydrates are the problem, and not fat. This was ignored by Ancel Keys, the American Heart Association, the US Department of Agriculture, the National Association of Heart, Lung, and Blood Institute, AMA, the McGovern Commission, and many other scientists. The American Heart Association received a lot of money from Procter & Gamble, and in return they offered an endorsement with their heart label on fatty products like lard and Crisco.

That cancer might be caused by sugar and carbohydrates in modern diets was of concern to doctors working with primitive populations. Cancer started appearing when these populations started eating the Western diet. From the Arctic to Africa, scientists followed the transition from ancient diets to Western diets of sugar and carbohydrates. Whenever people started eating the Western diet, they developed heart disease, diabetes, and cancer. This was an epidemic studied by many scientists.

A German doctor named Otto Schaefer visited the well-known Inuit tribe, studied by many scientists, in the Canadian Arctic in 1951. He was on Baffin Island, where there was no Western food and a very low level of Western diseases.

The Hudson Bay Company began bringing in loads of Western food, including flour and molasses. Some communities ate this, and others didn't get any of this type of food. This gave Dr. Schaefer an opportunity to study the same culture's reaction to different ways of eating. The Inuit who ate the ancient way remained very healthy. The ones who ate the Western way became sick.

What was hard to understand was that on their old diet, in spite of eating very few vegetables and having very little sunshine, they had no deficiencies of any vitamins, including vitamin D, vitamin C, and other multivitamins. That has been very difficult to explain. Whenever the natives stopped eating meat, they replaced it with sugar and carbohydrates. Dr. Schaefer observed that the natives eating large amounts of sugar changed their health greatly over a twenty-year period. Dr. Schaefer told a local newspaper, "It was self-inflicted genocide." Dr. Yudkin, who wrote *Pure, White and Deadly*, claimed that a twenty-year lag is typical of the time it takes for the Western chronic diseases to appear. I personally think that the lag time is a lot shorter than that. For many people, thirty days of nothing but fast food could make them diabetic.

The British Royal Navy surgeon Captain Thomas Cleve saw some of the same phenomena in many remote areas to which he was transferred in the early 1900s. He called the chronic disease "saccharine disease" and wrote a famous book later by that name. I highly recommend reading it. I wonder whether Dr. Ancel Keys or the scientists at the American Heart Association, NIH, or the American Association of Heart, Lung, and Blood Institute ever read that book.

Boatloads of sugar came to the British Isles in the 1670s. The slave trade was started over sugar. It didn't stop until the 1850s. People in Britain consumed about four pounds of sugar per year in 1670, which increased to twenty pounds in the 1800s and now is about 180 pounds a year, as in the United States—about half a pound a day.

Heart disease began to appear in the mid-1800s, and it was thought that meant that sugar was the answer. Meat consumption stayed the same, but heart disease increased after that. The only element of the diet to keep pace with heart disease was sugar. Fat consumption stayed the same. Then Banting came along with his story and book. Rates of cancer also increased dramatically. Cancer went from being a rarity and essentially unknown in the Eskimos and Indian tribes. We all know now cancer is a sugar-feeder. Seventy percent of uterine cancer occurs in overweight people, and about 30 percent of breast cancers are related to the estrogen in fat.

SUGAR

Sugar is our cocaine. We are hardwired for sweets by evolution. All our survival instincts, such as sex and eating, are attached to pleasure by chemistry. Sugar makes us feel great and is addictive.

The taste buds for sugar are located throughout the mouth, tongue, hard palate, and soft palate and down the esophagus to the stomach, and even beyond to the pancreas and bowel. Sugar receptors have been found throughout this region. The receptors are not located just on the tip of the tongue, as some people might want you to think. We have taste buds for salt, sugar, bitter, and sour and appreciate the softness and palatability of fat, although no receptors have been found for fat. It is thought that there is a sense of taste for meat products, called umami. We have thousands of taste bud receptors for sugar, and they're hooked to the brain, the pleasure center.

As you know, sugar is in a lot of our drinks, causing at least one-half of the obesity epidemic, and is an ingredient in 80 percent of all sixty thousand food products. Our sugar comes from three products: cane sugar, sugar beets, and corn.

Christopher Columbus brought sugar to the New World, and it was planted in Santo Domingo. The Germans discovered in the 1700s that you could extract glucose from beets. During wartime, people in France realized you could extract sugar from beets, and now it's grown that way all over the world. Beets were the main source of sugar till around 1970. Then the Japanese invented high-fructose corn syrup, HFCS, which is much sweeter and cheaper than sugar and became very popular in the industry quickly. One of the reasons that it's cheaper is because the US government subsidizes corn.

Unfortunately, corn syrup is high in fructose, which is metabolized not in the bloodstream but in the liver and made into low-density LDL, the one that doesn't float but burrows its way into the blood vessels, neural cells, and so on; it also has a lot to do with arthritis and hypertension.

In the 1960s it was proven in lab rats that sugar is addictive. Graduate student Anthony Scalafani studied the effectiveness of sugar and fat with functional MRI scans. The brain just lit up. He published a paper in 1976 with experimental proof of food craving as an addiction.

In Philadelphia there is a place called the Monell Chemical Senses Center, which is supported 50 percent by the government and 50 percent by the food industry. Guess who has a lot of influence there. They found and discovered a blood protein that is on the taste buds for sugar. That's how they were able to trace the tremendous distribution of sugar taste buds throughout the mouth, esophagus, and gut.

They also determined that children and African Americans are particularly keen on foods that are salty and sweet. The marketing people have taken full advantage of that. Hypertension is particularly high in the African American population, so salt intake turns out to be something they really have to watch. When I worked as a resident in neurosurgery in Washington, DC, I treated a lot of brain hemorrhages from hypertension in the black population. I saw blood pressures that were so high that I've never seen them again, fortunately.

At the Monell Institute, they proved that children were actually becoming addicted to sugar because they were developing a tolerance for sugar. In other words, you have to keep on increasing the amount, just like a narcotic addict, to get the same effect. It's the taste, the flavor, the sensation, and the psychological satisfaction that they are looking for. Babies are born with taste buds for sugar, and it's based on their biology, it's based on evolution, and it's important for the survival.

A man named Moscowitz from White Plains, New York, whose company dealt with product development related to food substances and chemicals, did his best work with sugar. He used mathematical calculations to create the biggest craving. Moscowitz worked on "optimal sensory linking." Hunger was found to be a poor driver of cravings. Emotional needs are more important.

Taste, aroma, appearance and texture are very important.

The convenience of fast-food restaurants brought the fat and sugar chemicals to the forefront of the etiology of obesity. The "cocaine effect" of sugar is its mother and father. The king is sugar because of fructose. Convenient, fast, and addictive, salt and sugar drive the car. That process has been experimentally, chemically, and mathematically proven. Look at the result: America is the land of obesity.

It all started at the beginning of the last century. John Harvey Kellogg took over a health facility in Battle Creek, Michigan. The popular diagnosis at that time was neurasthenia, and he ran a four-hundred-bed hospital or institute. He came back from a trip to Colorado with an idea to create a breakfast cereal from corn. His brother Will, an accountant, managed to figure out how to make the cereal sweeter, and the rest is history. Fat-laden breakfast foods of the 1900s were then replaced by the sugar-laden cereals of the twentieth century, and we've all seen the result. Kellogg was home to 108 brands of cereal, and he then developed his own company doing the same thing. Kellogg was composed of the top players for a long time. The FDA was in bed with these companies and didn't consider sugar a threat to our health.

Dr. Jean Mayer, a Harvard professor, has called obesity the disease of civilization. He discovered that the desire to eat is controlled by the hypothalamus in the brain.

Advertising to small children by food companies became rampant. It was outlawed in European countries. We restricted it only up to age eleven after a long fight, but companies simply increased advertisements to teenagers, and sales were not affected much.

Robert Woodruff, the CEO of Coca-Cola, had two brilliant but deadly innovations. In 1927 he introduced Coca-Cola with its sugary drinks to the rest of the world; in World War II, any soldier anywhere in the world could get a Coke for five cents. I suspect he addicted the whole bunch. He figured out how to get to people's emotions with sugar.

A man named Jeffrey Dunn became head of the South American division of Coca-Cola; in 2001 he visited Brazil looking for new territory. He was looking at poor neighborhoods for potential sales. He woke up and said, "I'm not going to do this." He decided the company went too far. Guess what? He no longer worked for Coca-Cola after that trip.

The Coke and Pepsi war has sugar as its king, with coffee not far behind.

In 1981 Coca-Cola switched to high-fructose corn syrup because it was cheaper and sweeter; when it studied its customer base, it didn't speak about loyal customers but called them heavy users, as one would speak about drug addicts.

Eighty percent of the world's sugar is consumed by 20 percent of the people.

Nestlé, Kraft, Coke, and Pepsi all decreased the size of their drinks for a while so they could charge less and increase sales, especially in countries like Brazil. It's called the elasticity of demand. I see it demonstrated at my gym, and it works. They have nine thousand members where I work out, ten dollars a month; I compliment them every day. A lot of people are getting in shape there. What they don't realize, though, is exercise is only about 25 percent of it.

I noticed in the news that Mexico may be passing a law putting a 10 percent tax on sugars and soda and 8 percent on fast food. Hallelujah to that.

In 1964, a man named John Yudkin published a book in Britain called *Pure, White and Deadly*. He also published countless papers on the biochemistry of sucrose. Remember, sucrose is 50 percent glucose, 50 percent fructose. Fructose gives the sweetness and is metabolized by the liver and converted to low-density cholesterol, small LDL fragments that penetrate the blood vessels and cause atherosclerosis and a number of other illnesses. It's clearly a toxin and is associated with vascular disease, heart disease, stroke, and other inflammatory illnesses.

Ancel Keys, an epidemiologist from Minnesota, invented the K-rations used during World War II. However, people started to note that high-fat dishes were leading to a high rate of vascular disease. This resulted in a battle between the fat and sugar camps as to the cause of disease. In 1970, Michael Brown and Joseph Goldstein in Dallas discovered HDL and LDL cholesterol and described the LDL receptor. This was a very important discovery. They correlated LDL cholesterol with coronary heart disease. Then we followed through with a national low-fat diet recommendation and forgot about the sugar.

Senator George McGovern appointed a reporter named Nick Mottern with no scientific background to research and write a paper called "The Dietary Goals for the United States." He gathered information from the work of Mark Hegsted, a nutritionist at Harvard. The latter thought that saturated fat was the cause of our health problems. The USDA, the American Heart Association, and the Society of Clinical Nutritionists all endorsed the document. The industry responded with low-fat, high-sugar products, and you can see the result. A very obese nation became worse.

The mistake was in assuming that all LDL was bad; it turns out there are two types of LDL, A and B. As already mentioned, the large LDL floats in the blood vessels and represents 80 percent of it. Of the small LDL, 20 percent is produced in the liver from glucose and fructose, not fat.

A nurses' health study followed fifty thousand postmenopausal nurses and fed them a diet that was either 30 percent or 40 percent fat, and they found no difference in the incidence of vascular disease. I've heard others say that they didn't drop the fat percentage low enough, and that's a justifiable criticism. Dr. Joel Fuhrman said they should've dropped it to 20 percent, and the results would have been different.

The food industry took the fat out. The food tasted like cardboard, and they solved that problem quickly by adding a lot of sugar. Sales went up tremendously, the industry was very happy, and the country became sick. Our federal government supported the price of corn, wheat, and rye. In the 1990s more low-fiber and high-sugar foods were produced. The obesity epidemic was born. Seemingly logical, well-meaning people who don't understand the biochemistry of food have made a lot of people sick and continue to do so.

Our bodies have not adjusted to all of this sugar, especially fructose, and it's killing us; we consume 60 pounds of fructose a year, 33 pounds of high-fat cheese, and 150 pounds of sugar. We are sugar and fat loaded; nobody and our bodies are revolting. It's become a public health problem, and the government needs to act.

Early Diagnosis

There is a lot of controversy here. Opinion, frankly, carries the day. Decades-old double-blind studies of nutrition and eating habits are hard to find. Forty-four years of experience in the field should have some value.

Common sense is king here. The HRA, health risk assessment, should be number one. That should begin in childhood. At exactly what age? That would depend on family history and whether the child has an unusual early onset of obesity. If the grandparents, siblings, or mother or father has significant metabolic illnesses or death at a young age, then biometric and blood tests should be run as early as age two. The rate of obesity is actually accelerating in the two- to six-year-old age range. The sooner you correct the problem, the easier it will be. Eating habits honestly become more difficult to correct the longer they have been there.

Blood work will generally be abnormal before obesity sets in, but not always. Children should have their weight and height checked at least once a year and more often with a strong family history. If both parents are overweight, then the child has a 70 percent chance of being overweight. If one parent has a weight problem, then it runs around 30 to 40 percent. Generally, many providers don't check the biometrics or the blood work of teenagers unless there is a strong family history of chronic disease. Personally, I think that is a mistake. Even if they have a normal BMI, teens should fill out an HRA form and have their biometrics checked. After all, we're looking to reduce the rate of this plague tremendously. In the long run, it will prevent a tremendous amount of illness and save a tremendous amount of healthcare dollars.

You need to check the metabolism of the liver after a basic HRA, including the following:

- NMR-lipid profile: This determines the particle size and number of LDL, HDL, and triglycerides. Large amounts of small dense LDL are a sign of trouble. Even normal cholesterol won't tell the story. You need a low-density LDL test. You should have fewer than one thousand LDL particles and fewer than five hundred small LDL particles.
- Liver enzyme tests—AST, ALT, GGT—to assess fatty liver
- Two-hour glucose-tolerance test
- Serum insulin and blood sugar (one to two hours of fasting)
- Lipid profile
- Cholesterol: <150
- LDL: <70
- HDL: >60—female
- HDL: >50—male
- Triglycerides: <100
- Triglyceride/HDL ratio
- Total cholesterol/HDL ratio
- Hemoglobin A1c
- Gluten panel sensitivity test

An insulin-response test is very important to catch early metabolic syndrome or type 2 diabetes. This test measures your insulin and blood sugar at the same time. This will help providers catch the majority of metabolic diseases very early, when it is much easier to correct them. The test measures glucose and insulin levels after a seventy-five-gram gross load. Your blood sugar can be normal, but you insulin could be sky high. I saw this many times in my practice. That is why diabesity, the co-occurrence of diabetes and obesity, is not diagnosed early in 90 percent of people who have it. You can see why this is so critical. Look at the tremendous amount of disease we misdiagnose.

If you have abnormal lab tests, they should be repeated at least every three months while you are taking corrective action. The provider should see you frequently; otherwise, get a new provider or insist on more-frequent tests. To assess the severity of complications, if you have an abnormal metabolic test and it is clear you have a problem, you need to get additional blood tests. If you would like to use the Internet, take advantage of Dr. Mark Hyman's excellent website. I also recommend his book *The Blood Sugar Solution*. You can download it at www.bloodsugarsolution.drhyman. com.

If we are going to stop this epidemic, we need to start very early. Not everyone would agree. If 20 to 40 percent of people with normal weight have abnormal biometric liver testing, then according to Dr. Mark Hyman, we need to do regular biometric testing. This is the future. It is a lot easier to take corrective action at a young age. If we miss disease for up to a decade, then that person is missing out on years of his or her life. We spend $2.7 trillion on healthcare yearly; we could reduce this by $1 trillion if we take more early action. Right now, instead of healthcare, we have "sick care." Obese teenagers should be treated aggressively while we still have a chance to change their habits. Everyone should exercise at least thirty minutes per day.

Although we don't hear a lot of great things about the English healthcare system, they practice preventative healthcare big time. Almost all patients have their biometrics tested on a yearly basis because it has been found to be highly preventative. Doctors' offices are full of signs promoting wellness with phone numbers to call for additional help. Family doctors get paid more for keeping patients well. You will notice when you travel in Europe that obesity is not much of a problem. When Europeans come here, they are shocked by the size of our population. We badly need to create a culture of wellness, and number one in that paradigm is that the patient must participate in his or her healthcare. In addition, providers need to participate by teaching every patient when the opportunity arises. For example, I have CDs, DVDs, and TV shows and take the time to coach most patients in spite of a very busy schedule. I've been doing this for more than thirty years. I also write books, and they're all on Amazon. The majority are about wellness from every angle.

In summary, I highly recommend really persistent, repeated HRA and biometric testing as the best way to turn the US healthcare crisis around.

Motivation and Breathing

Many breathing techniques lead to wellness. The ancient Chinese, the Taoist, and the Hindu yoga traditions use breathing techniques extensively to achieve a quiet state of mindfulness. This leads to good health and stress reduction.

The Buddha gave simple instructions that form the basis for breath meditation. The meditator assumes the lotus position, a cross-legged posture. The only time that mindfulness can happen is in the present moment; if you think you know the past, that is memory. Mindfulness is unbiased. It is not for or against anything. When you focus on the breath for a few moments, your thinking calms itself. Therefore, you could be doing anything—walking, combing your hair, doing the dishes; if you are concentrating on your breath, this will lead to mindfulness. It's meditation.

When we focus on the breath, we are focusing on the life-force. Life begins with the first breath and will end after our last. To contemplate breathing is to contemplate life itself. Ancient India had a tremendous respect for the breath, a deep understanding of its powerful effect on the body and mind. In fact, all of the Indian spiritual sciences had some form of *pranayama*, which is usually translated as "breath control." Most forms of pranayama, yogic breathing, involve controlling the breath. The quality of the breathing does improve; it becomes fuller, freer, and calmer, with consequences both physical and psychological. We're all breathing. We need to be aware of the simple sensation, the in breath and the out breath. We note that a deep breath relaxes the body and figure that an accomplished meditator will be breathing deeply all the time, period. If we allow the breath to unfold naturally, without tampering with it, in time we may be able to do that with other aspects of our experience; we might learn to let the feelings be, let the mind be. Using meditation in its extreme form allows you to develop a Zen mind. The ultimate goal, the Zen mind is not easy to achieve and takes time to develop.

The breath is an ideal vehicle for teaching Buddhism in the West. It is not religion. It's a way of being, a mindful way of life that leads to wellness. For some people, breathing it isn't a terribly pleasant process. A lifetime of faulty breathing, often accompanied by emotional blockages, has made the breath an unattractive object of attention. You need to develop a certain devotion to your meditation, such as counting to ten or repeating the same word to quiet the mind, in combination with the breathing techniques. Pick a time of day in a quiet place; it could be anywhere. You can meditate sitting at the stoplight or cleaning the toilet.

An excellent way to relax is to concentrate on the breath when taking a walk. It's meditative and leads to healing of the stressful mind. At the beginning and at the end of a walk, stand and breathe mindfully for a few moments. Pay attention to every aspect of breathing, the nose, the lungs, the diaphragm, and the abdomen. Breathe like a baby, so the belly hangs out when you breathe in deeply. Pay attention to every part of your body and your surroundings—this is meditation.

Saint Francis of Assisi said, "It is no use walking anywhere to preach unless our walking is our preaching." There are five rewards for one who practices walking meditation: you can endure traveling by foot, you can endure exertion, you become free from disease, whatever you have eaten and drunk becomes well digested, and the concentration you win while doing walking meditation lasts a long time. It's this concentration, and the joy of walking in such a state, that is the primary reward, and a state of wellness is close behind.

Sometimes the breath is very fine, like silk or satin; it enters and exits freely. And other times it is coarse, more like burlap, and fights it's way in and out. Sometimes the breath is so deep in its root that it affects the whole body, relaxing it profoundly. As you pay attention to breathing, the quality of the breathing changes, perhaps because thinking is diminished. The breath becomes deeper, you find it more enjoyable, and the body starts to reap the fruits of that, to become more relaxed.

It just reflects the power of mindfulness. If your mind becomes angry, all worried, your heart starts to race, and your body grows tense. But if you can just be with the breath for a while, not suppressing the emotion but agreeing with it, all changes. The mind becomes calm. As the breath goes, so goes the body. The first law of Buddhism is that everything is constantly changing. So your breathing technique can change from time to time. Breathing leaves all the troubles behind, all the preoccupations, worries, plans, doubts, fears, all the stuff that makes up the mind. Especially in the modern world, where everybody is so impressed with variety and complexity, so desperate to be entertained, it is a relief to settle into the simple repetitive act. The opportunity we have of staying with the breathing, consciously coming back to it, is a chance to do one simple, ordinary thing well. Entry into the spirit of repetition can be a powerful lesson in simplicity, which is desperately needed in the modern world. Many people come to meditation expecting some complex practice leading to an ordinary experience. They can't believe they're just supposed to sit there and watch the breath. We begin to see how useful the skill is in other aspects of our lives. The constant repetition of going back to the breath has real value. In some ways, this entire practice is everything the Buddha said, is concerned with having an infinite respect for life. The practice of breathing and meditation constantly reminds us that everything is worthy of attention. To be mindful of anything is an act of generosity. You are giving it life by allowing it into your world. But the greatest benefit is that you respect for your own life.

The breath is a vital conditioner of the body. The body, mind, and breath become one, and you are able to sit for a long time without pain or discomfort. It's important to emphasize that this process unfolds in different ways for different people, that it generally takes place over a long period of time, that for all, or most, of us it is the fruit of a great deal of sitting. It will cause us, though, to pay much more attention to what we are doing and get rid of destructive behaviors such as overeating, lack of exercise, smoking, drinking, and using drugs. All of the Buddha's teachings, it has been said, can be reduced to one: under no circumstances attach to anything as me or mine. It isn't that we shouldn't experience rapture or happiness, but we have to be careful not to attach anything to them.

A huge amount of fear, anxiety, and apprehension is stimulated by thought itself. That is what you are trying to avoid by paying attention to the breath and developing relaxing mindfulness. A usual reaction to fear is to create a battlefield. Our fear is that war, with our tremendous yearning to be free from it, and the state of battle is the mind and the body in which the process is taking place. We tie ourselves into knots, turn ourselves inside out, fighting that battle. The attitude of practice is to open the process up, to see that it's all part of us, the fear, the yearning to be free of it, the mind and the body, the mindfulness observing them, the conscious breathing that nurtures the mindfulness. We sit there with all of that, all one thing. Then one day it comes up; our attention meets it, becomes one with it, allows it to blossom, which is what the fear wanted all along, and then we can get rid of it. It is when we prevent the blossoming of fear by ignoring its presence that fear hangs around, drags us down, because we spend so much energy holding it off. Even in the blossom, life has its parts. That way, we have all the energy we would have used escaping it to combat it. We also have the energy of the fear itself. It is a great gain in energy when we let things happen. The ground of fearlessness is fear. In order to become fearless, you have to stand in the middle of your fear. We shouldn't trust any fearlessness that doesn't have that as its basis. The beginning of that is to see your fear and admit to it. You acknowledge that you are afraid, and then have the immense courage and humility to study it. It can be the beginning of the end of it. In other words, make a plan to get rid of it. Don't try to suppress it.

Mindfulness and breathing techniques are the road to freedom of the mind. The process of breathing shows us a way to let go of the old and be open to the new. The process of reading is a living metaphor for understanding how to expand our narrow sense of ourselves and to be present to the healing energies that are both in and around us. Some people say that the diaphragm is the "spiritual muscle." It lies at the foundation of healthy breathing. Shaped like a large dome, the diaphragm functions as both the floor of the chest cavity and the ceiling, all the abdominal cavity. When we inhale, the diaphragm normally contracts. This pump-like motion creates a partial vacuum, which, as you know, draws air into the lungs. When we inhale fully, the diaphragm can double or even triple its range of movement and massage the stomach, liver, pancreas, intestines, and kidneys, promoting intestinal movement, blood and lymph flow, and the absorption of nutrients. The work of breathing starts with sensing the inner atmosphere of our organism, the basic emotional stance we take toward the world and ourselves.

Learning how to observe the mechanism involved in breathing, as well as the various physical, emotional, and mental forces acting on them, depends in large part on learning how to sense ourselves, to listen to ourselves, to expand our attention to include the sensory impressions constantly arising in our organism. We have to learn to listen to our body.

Our Frontal Lobe Is in Charge and Motivates Us

One way or another, we are the ones who will make the decision on what to eat. We are the authors of our own health. We are the driver of that tank that is involved with this war of eating.

Women have more eating problems than men because they are in charge more often of buying food and preparing meals, and they face a constant barrage from the media and magazines about body size. Can you imagine buying food for a husband, yourself, and your children, who all have different appetites and food preferences, and trying to control the situation? The husband may have "inflexible palate syndrome" and just will not change what he eats in spite of being diabetic or a heart patient. He might say, "I can't possibly live without eating meat every day." The children are screaming out for sugary, fatty, and salty foods.

I would say with children it's a bit easier, because they will get hungry and you are buying the food. If there is a problem and your children are overweight, have an honest look at them. Don't deny the picture; bring in changes slowly, and they may not notice it. Their tastes will change. I slowly introduced a lot of vegetarian food at the doctors' lounge in the hospital. Frankly, they did not notice it, and the food looks great now. The dietitian is a friend of mine. Next week she's bringing in edamame on a regular basis. Sooner or later, the children's tastes will change. Educate them about school food, how to read labels, and how to avoid sugary drinks. The husband could be more of a problem. He may need to be educated about healthy food. Believe me, in my forty-five years of being a physician, I have seen that Americans in general eat the mad, toxic, sad foods, all fat, sugar, and salt—the killer triad of Americans.

Limiting your own or family members' food intake is like a starvation diet; it will not work and will result in overeating and snacking. Preparing food yourself on a daily basis makes it a lot more difficult, and quite easy to feed your own psychology with food. The food that causes the flow of dopamine is in your hands, a very tempting situation. Besides, you may be hungry. You look at food every day, making the meals and testing your self-control daily and sometimes multiple times a day. It is difficult for many. Family members may use food to control each other socially. One never eats; another overeats. One is perfect, and another is out of control. If you are overweight, people think that you're out of control, that you have emotional problems. Thinness is considered being in control, but many times it is not. Society looks at people with a normal weight as being in control of their lives. Body size is related to social stigma.

Over controlling behavior with food is a central problem with eating disorders, anorexia and bulimia. Eating control is thought to be the solution to obesity, but the answer to me is much more the type of food you are eating. If you're eating the correct food, control will follow. If you are eating a highly nutrient-dense food pattern, in general, you do not need even to watch your portions. Most of the time, it is difficult for us to have perfect control of our eating habits. I say food selection should lead the way to good health and proper weight.

You'll get some families like the one I saw last week, gathered around the table at a Japanese restaurant, where I clearly saw them all, twenty feet in front of me, from three-year-olds to eighty-year-olds, about ten of them, all seriously overweight. Children with puffy cheeks, adults with bellies hanging down, men and women—it was a sad sight. I would say odds are they totally blind to their situation—just like an anorexic.

How did this happen? Genetics accounts for only 20 percent. They're probably like many anorexic and overweight people; they don't see it in themselves. You do not see the potential health problems, and that is frankly all I'm talking about. I don't care about their appearance; many of these people are beautiful. I passionately care about their future of diabetes, heart disease and stroke, arthritis, dementia, and cancer. Their psychiatric needs and eating behavior probably are the same throughout the family; the anxiety and the lack of serotonin to feel good are about the same. Instead of using a tranquilizer, they are using food to feel good. They have a similar way of cooking, eat the same type of food, and most likely lack proper eating education. I would bet two or three already have diabetes, maybe one of them even as a teenager. I would bet everything I own that the two or three diabetics do not know that their type 2 diabetes is curable by getting down to a normal weight.

Food preferences are transmitted within the family from parent to child. Pleasurable fatty and sugary food chemically decreases anxiety and increases love. It's the womb, that caves, and escape from life's problems. The poor have this need more commonly, of course. That is the reason they have a much higher rate of overweight and obesity. Many times it's their only daily pleasure. There is much more obesity in the economically distressed. Food is also used among family members to distribute power and rewards and to control behavior. Eating behavior is used many times among family members to assume power and control. Eating behavior can keep the family together: to hell with the rest of the world, this is us!

An individual's thoughts and beliefs and attitudes greatly affect what he or she eats. Many people justify their food choices with incorrect information they obtain from some ineffective diet book. Many of the diet books are complete frauds. Individuals have a range of beliefs about the meaning of the food system and body size and shape. Many believe diets are all or nothing, and give up too easily.

Food deprivation will lead to overeating. High-protein diets don't work. Starving yourself of carbohydrates will sooner or later lead to overeating. Negative beliefs about obesity may motivate some people to achieve a normal weight—they don't want to look this way—and they become motivated to change. It's a complex psychological situation between the pleasure of eating and subsequent guilt.

As we know, women are the main providers of food in the family. Gender is central to many of the conflicts surrounding food. Eighty percent of the clients in my eating classes are female. There are a number of reasons for that. They also choose education about proper eating more commonly. Men don't want to give up that steak and would rather exercise. Women are treated differently in the media. You have to be thin to be on TV, although we have witnessed the yo-yo diets of Oprah. I suspect that situation is all about psychology. Women show more body dissatisfaction than men, and body size is also more important to women's self-esteem. Most anorexics and bulimics are women. Abdominal fat is more dangerous, and men have more of that; female fat is usually around the buttocks and thighs.

Food choice is affected by social norms. Certain ethnic groups make better or worse food choices. The famous China study by Dr. T. Colin Campbell, where researchers studied Chinese people and related eating patterns. In other cultures, overweight and obesity is rampant in more than 50 percent of the people, and those cultures have diabetes and its consequences. Family and cultural norms affect our image of ourselves. Certain ethnic groups accept obesity.

Dieting, not food selection is the media's choice to lose weight. This sells diet books, but they usually don't work. They're not concerned since they already made the money.

Social norms of attractiveness contribute to the discrimination against and stereotyping of those who are overweight and obese. Peer influence and social support can be used to modify eating behavior in the overweight. And this is a socially desirable state, which can lead to eating disorders. The psychological effects of the chemicals of food—dopamine, serotonin, endorphins, and beta-endorphins—probably are the great drivers of food choices and habits.

The individual, the family, and the group have great effects on the food choices that we make. Some ethnic groups think cheese is everything, although, mind you, it's 80 percent fat.

We have to eat every day, so the cue is there continuously; the lack of serotonin cries out for relief. It is a combination of stress relief, exercise, and food choice that will lead to proper eating habits and good health. You are the author of your health! Fat, sugar, and salt are nasty chemicals that lead to being overweight and obese. Good luck in your choices.

VISUALIZATION

Visualization is the language of the subconscious mind; in essence, it is how we speak to the brain. If we create an image of what we would like to achieve, it is more likely to happen. Your brain will not be able to differentiate between what is real and what is not when you speak to it in pictures and images. It can be very motivating and brings your thoughts into action. The human body contains about seventy trillion cells, and by creating images, you are motivating these cells into action.

How does visualization work? Our bodies in the universe are essentially composed of energy. A thought is a quick and mobile force of energy. When we create or accomplish something, we always do it first by using our thought process. Thinking precedes action. Any image creates energy, and having an idea, picture, or thought tends to attract and create that energy form in reality. We are always attracting the energy of life—whatever we think about the most, believe in the most, or are able to visualize most vividly. When you visualize your goal, it is much more likely to happen because the act of creating images, or visualization, immobilizes and motivates your seventy trillion plus body cells into action.

Visualization works best after a period of meditation and deep breathing. While sitting in the yoga position or sitting in a chair, take about ten to twenty deep abdominal breaths and create a picture of your goal. Use all of your senses—smells, feelings, tastes, sounds, and detailed pictures. Do it frequently. If you are visualizing weight loss, picture yourself on the beach during the morning sunrise, wearing great workout clothes, ready to go. Begin your stretch while you smell the ocean air, hear the waves, and feel the warmth of the sun energizing your body. Start your stretching, and visualize yourself taking off on a beautiful morning run down the shore. Or imagine that new car, house, or career. You may even imagine doing missionary work and the great feeling it gives you.

When you have the image in your mind, make some affirmative statements to yourself, silently or out loud. "I'm going to lose those thirty pounds; I will have that great job; I will stop smoking; I will stop drinking; I will stop taking so many medications; I will cure my type 2 diabetes with proper eating." There are no limits to what you can accomplish through the use of imagery and visualization! The more frequently you do this, and the more detail you give to using your five senses, the most likely you are to achieve your goal. Affirmative statements are very motivating.

Learn to use meditation or deep breathing first so that you are in a relaxed state. This destresses your body, and you will see the images more clearly. And you are more likely to achieve your goal as you relax each muscle in your body. Count backward from twenty—this is a mantra that will lead you into a meditative state. Meditation and visualization will relax you and renew your spirit and can be used anytime during the day.

Imagery is a powerful and mysterious force in human nature that is able to bring about dramatic improvement in our lives. It is a kind of mental engineering that works best when supported by meditation, and especially strong religious faith. It is not difficult to practice, and anyone can do it. It has caught the attention of doctors, psychologists, and "thinkers" everywhere. The word "imagine" is derived from imagination. Imagery, utilizing the feeling of mental pictures or images, is based on the principle that there is a deep tendency in human nature to become precisely like that which we imagine ourselves to be. An image formed and held tenaciously in the conscious mind passes the present state by mental osmosis and travels into the unconscious mind. Once accepted firmly in the unconscious state, the individual strongly tends to grasp it, and it then becomes part of the individual. The imagery effect on thought and performance is so powerful that a long-held vision of an objective or goal could become determinative.

Imaging is positive thinking. Carry this state one step further, and you could say that imaging is a laser beam of the imagination, a shaft of mental energy, in which the desired goal or outcome is pictured so vividly by the conscious mind that the unconscious mind accepts it and is activated by it. This release is so powerful in total force that it can bring about astonishing changes in the life of the person who is doing the imaging.

Let me give you some examples. Jim Thorpe, a famous Olympic athlete, while traveling by boat to Europe never practiced with the athletes on the ship. He never stretched, lifted weights, or jogged. Instead, he sat in the corner, using imagery, about every Olympic event he was to participate in. And he won almost every track event! He had the used the power of imagery. My racecar friend, John Burton, whom I play tennis with in Florida, once told me a story. Many of the famous racecar drivers imagine the event the night before, using imagery to successfully carry out their goals. Additionally, during the Vietnam War, an imprisoned sergeant, Sergeant Gordon, visualized playing eighteen holes of golf every day for seven years. When he was released from prison, during his first game in the United States, he shot the best score of his life! That's the power of visualization.

The anticipatory power of the imagination has been utilized in many sports, and scientific research has established its effectiveness for athletes. This research shows that by picturing the successful completion of moves they want to make, athletes can improve their performance—especially if the mental picture is accompanied with physical practice. Good athletes have physical and mental self-control. Jack Nicklaus, author of *Golf My Way*, claimed that hitting a good shot depends 10 percent on swing mechanics, 40 percent on set up and stance, and 50 percent on his mental picture. In his book he describes how to visualize a shot before he makes it; he describes it like making a very colorful movie. He never hits the shot, even in practice, without having a very sharp and focused picture of it in his head. First, he sees the ball, nice and white and sitting up high on the bright green grass. Then the scene quickly changes, and he sees the ball getting to where he wants it—its path, its trajectory and shape, even its behavior on the landing. Just make your movie that shows a perfect shot. I always visualize my serve while playing tennis. And other athletes use this power all the time also. In sports, great athletes visualize what they wish to do, practice the living daylights out of it, and then they don't think when they play the sport; it has now become automatic.

There are four basic steps for effective visualization: set your goal by tweaking a clear idea or picture, enhance this goal by using the five senses, focus on the goal often, and give yourself positive energy with affirmations of achieving this goal.

For many people, affirmations are most powerful and inspiring when they include references to a spiritual source. There are three elements within you that determine how to successfully create what will work for you in any given situation: desire, belief, and acceptance. These define your intention. Your spiritual source is a supply of infinite love, wisdom, and energy in the universe. Continue to practice your relaxation, visualization, and affirmations daily.

Healing conscious creative visualization is a process of creating positive thoughts and images to communicate with our bodies—to remove our thoughts out of a place of negativity to a place of positivity, and to replace constrictive and what may be literally sickening thoughts with positive energy.

One can also use visualization and imaging to treat cancer. Dr. Carl Simington published a great book called *Getting Well Again*. In this book, he describes great visualization techniques to destroy cancer cells. If cancer is your problem, this is a great book to read. It has helped a lot of cancer patients. Imaging can also be used to help your pain problems. As a neurosurgeon, I have had a lot of experience with this, and it can be very helpful.

Imagery and healing is probably best known for its direct effects on your own physiology. Through imagery, you can stimulate changes in many bodily functions usually considered inaccessible by a conscious influence. Imagery is a natural language of a major part of our nervous system. It has been shown that the two sides of the human brain think in very different ways. They are simultaneously capable of independent thought. The left and right sides of the brain are different. The right side of the brain speaks in images; the left side of brain speaks more in terms of language and numbers. This essential difference between the two parts of the brains is a relatively new way of thinking. The left-brain processes information sequentially, while the right brain processes it simultaneously and specifically.

Everyday-life imagery has been presented as a powerful device to achieve major goals and objectives. Use it every day. It can be used to smooth out the minor wrinkles of living. Many famous inventions were produced by the use of imagery. Imagery has its own formula: the goal, purpose, prayer activity, thoughtful planning, innovative thinking, organization, hard work, and always holding the image of success firmly in mind. If this process is faithfully carried out, the desired results will be achieved, despite any and all difficulties or setbacks.

You Can If You Think You Can

If you have a wellness problem, now or in the future, you come to the realization something needs to be done. Maybe it's obesity, vascular disease with strokes and heart attacks, or type 2 diabetes. Don't feel hopeless or give up; do something about it. Anything is possible. Even if it's advanced cancer, positive thinking and mind-body techniques can double your lifespan and increase the spontaneous-cure rate—based on my own experience and what I have read in the literature. Cancer specialists as a group are just too pessimistic. There are so many books on the subject. They fill my library, books on hope and what to do.

When you have a problem, one that is especially difficult and baffling, perhaps unendurable and discouraging, there is one basic principle—never quit. To do so is to admit defeat, and your defeatist attitude will come true. Giving up shows a defective personality. It tends to develop a defeatist psychology.

Come at the problem in a different way if the methodology you're using is not working. And if the new approach is not working, come at it yet another way until you find the key. The computer button that turns on the human brain, your mind, remembers what it is like to be well. Be persistent; it's always too soon to quit.

How do you develop this undefeatable attitude? You need to develop a program of hope. Throw hopelessness out the window. Don't talk yourself into defeat. It is dangerous to use negative words. "No" denotes that you shut the door. It means defeat; it delays improvement. Turn things around, and now you have more. Meet the problem. Change your thinking; meet the problem in a positive, constant optimistic way. Make a plan; write it down. It's motivating.

The refusal to quit is called the persistence principle. Perseverance will win the day—don't be a quitter. Send out your positive vision; you cannot create success anywhere in this life without this application of the persistence principle.

Keep thinking positively. Much rain wears down marble. I saw that myself at Saint Peter's Cathedral in Rome. If you don't first succeed, then try again. The perception of all of yourself is critical and is applied by the perseverance principle.

Many times we are our own worst enemy. People can have goals and objectives and work hard and still fail. Perhaps you need to look at yourself, and something is amiss in yourself. Sharing what you think may be your personality defects with another person, almost any person, can be of great value, especially if you bring spirituality into it. Remember, attending church is the path to spirituality, no matter what religion.

The hardest person to know is yourself. We have a built-in self-protecting mechanism that always tries to do what we want. It seeks to make the irrational appear rational. Many people will talk about other people and their problems, but they hide from themselves and their own problems.

People fail usually do that, not because they unable to handle another situation—this is just in conflict with what they've been doing. Remember, if you're doing the same thing again and again, don't expect a different outcome.

You must see yourself as you really are and deal with yourself on that honest basis. That is the perception concept. And it is based on self-examination, taking a realistic look at yourself, because you're nearing the end of the road, or just traveling on the road of poor health and lack of wellness. Stand in front of a mirror, and say to yourself, "Now I want the truth about you."

Most people will realize that self-knowledge is always the beginning of self-development. The process is motivated by perception and releases new powers. It is the road that leads to successful achievement. Plugging away will win the day. Problems are a sign of life. Success weakens you; problem solving strengthens you.

How do you solve a problem and get motivated to solve the problem? If you acknowledge the problem, and apply thought and belief, then you have taken a long step down the road to handling it successfully.

Study your health problem, read about it, attend my free lectures, become knowledgeable, and then find the weak spot. Break the problem apart, and the rest will be easy. We need the body to carry the brain around. The mind is you. The tendency is to react emotionally rather than to think. The human mind will not think properly when it is hot. Cool it when problems start. Make use of your spiritual power. You can if you think you can, because all the ideas you need to handle every problem are all about you. Cool reactions will open up the lines of communication by which ideas flow to you. The chief duty of a human being is to master life.

To be healthy, vital, and alive, it is very important how you think. To a degree you can think yourself sick, or you can think yourself well. The soul becomes dyed with the color of its thoughts. If you think unhealthy, you will become unhealthy. Think defeat, and you will tend to create the circumstances that lead to defeat. You can if you think you can. In the matter of well-being, positive results come from visualizing yourself as whole, and you will act on it and get it done.

Food Addiction and Plain Overeating

A food craving can be powerful and irresistible, as we all know. Chocolate generates passion. Chocolate is the perfect food; it releases the feel-good chemicals. A binge eater can be addicted to fat, so a bag of potato chips can be consumed in no time flat. I saw it recently across the aisle in an airplane: a man, clearly overweight, opened a bag of potato chips—actually, he tore it open with his teeth—and this large bag was gone in three minutes. That same person may be bored eating a healthy whole-grain chip. It's the fat, salt, and sugar, our old friends.

Sometimes we think and obsess about food, planning, hoarding, sneaking, and hiding—just like an addict. Many of the original research studies on brain chemicals that regulate appetite have been reproduced, and the effect of chemicals on eating is well known. Some of us have mild addictions, and others can consume large amounts of any food. All of us can be helped to reverse this process by understanding the chemistry.

I listened this morning to the president's wife, whom I respect greatly, speak of childhood obesity. She seemed to say it's okay to eat all types of food. It gave me the impression that she did not realize how serious a problem childhood obesity is in the nation. It came across to me that she did not understand that food is a chemical and we need to change our psychology to make any progress on the problem. A lot of us need to practice abstinence from certain foods, or we will never lose that weight and avoid obesity and all the diseases that are associated with it. We must face the problem head-on, or we will continue on our merry way.

Food addiction in many ways is tougher than alcohol addiction, because we have to eat every day. We don't have to drink alcohol every day. Because of that, to change how we feel about food can be more difficult, and many times we don't know the composition of the food that we are eating. We must want to identify the trigger chemicals in our food. Small amounts of fatty, sugary, and salty food may not be addictive. Then again, a small amount of alcohol can start the process all over again. Then again, eating just one fatty potato chip can lead to the whole bag. One piece of chocolate, and we eat the whole box.

The recovery from eating bad food may be rapid; it can be done in thirty days. You can get rid of type II diabetes in thirty to sixty days. I have seen it in my proper eating classes and read about it many times in books. Understanding the brain chemistry of food and the practice of abstinence from certain foods can help us all. Your mind will be clear. You won't feel drugged anymore.

Addiction is deep dependence on a substance or activity to the extent that normal functioning is impaired. Food addiction is characterized by loss of control over eating. Physical dependence usually is related to certain type of food—it's the chemical effects on our brain cells.

Loss of control can be in regard to types of food chosen. Loss of control can be seen also in eating excessive quantities of food. Some people who overeat may even eat a balanced diet, but just eat two to three times as much as they should. Loss of control may be seen as eating at inappropriate times or in inappropriate places, such as hiding food in your desk at work or, yes, eating a chocolate bar while driving. Habituation to food means depending psychologically on the chemicals of food. We demonstrate psychological dependence when we are ready for something sweet. When you come home from work, as a reward for making it through this tough, stressful day, you need a fix, food or alcohol sometimes, unfortunately. It takes a war to stop that. Our first stresses in life as a baby are met with sugar or food. The bottle is given to stop our crying; our real need, cuddling, may not be met.

Food is probably used for psychological purposes more than any other substance. Food is a lifeline, an essential tool in our emotional survival kit. It takes us away from stress. It stops the world and lets us get off. It's a womb, a haven, a cave, an escape, and a refuge. Eating is an automatic response to feelings. To diminish the power of food can take a revolution. If food is removed, an equally strong force must replace it.

Physical dependence or addiction to a substance means the body has altered in some way that makes the absence of the substance painful. Addictive substances are used to mask pain. We have developed multiple receptor sites in our brain to adjust to the changing concentration of sugar, fat, and salt in our food. Our neurons and neurotransmitters have changed. This is a real physical adjustment in our brain. The extra receptor sites hurt if we don't supply the proper food chemicals. Our brain has changed. Frankly, it is no different from cocaine addiction, perhaps a little less intense. The thought of food produces dopamine; cocaine produces high levels of addictive dopamine. We can become addicted only to substances that out body already makes—interestingly, it is the presence of the new receptors on our neurons, which never go away, that makes readdiction to bad food so easy. It is no different from alcohol addiction. That's why alcoholics can't have even one drink.

Physical addiction occurs when neural functioning is altered as a result of eating high-fat, high-sugar foods. The addictive substance has altered the body and brain. You develop signs of physical addiction: an increasing tolerance to the food chemicals, and adaptation, so it takes more food to satisfy you. It takes a lot of food to make you feel better. Eating the substance, a strong indication of physical dependence, relieves the cycle of discomfort in withdrawal. This is a vicious cycle. Most people addicted to sugar or fat are also addicted to refined carbohydrates, which in essence are sugars. These foods have been stripped of their fiber content and are nothing but pure sugar. Food, drug, and alcohol addiction processes are very similar. Eating sugar is as good as a drink. They all alter the brain chemistry.

Two types of chemicals are involved with food addiction, serotonin and endorphin. Both are neural transmitters released from the ends of nerves (see illustration). They stimulate the next nerve, and the nerve impulse moves on. Serotonin promotes relaxation, peacefulness, and relief from pain, decreases anxiety, and in the end reduces the appetite. Endorphin is a neurotransmitter and your own body's morphine. It relieves pain and increases the sensation of pleasure. Breathing techniques and exercise, which reduces your appetite, can produce it. Both chemicals are highly concentrated in the hypothalamus, your brain's brain, and your metabolic center, the Wizard of Oz of the body. The hypothalamus regulates your appetite, sex, temperature, and a lot of the autonomic nervous system.

Perhaps people with food addiction or an overeating problem have a dysfunction of their serotonin levels. Something is missing in their lives, and food is the substitute. A person without serotonin will feel stress. When refined carbohydrates, sugar products, pasta, alcohol, and white bread are consumed, serotonin is released, and they feel better.

Certain endorphins and beta-endorphins stimulate the appetite. Overweight people have an increased beta-endorphin level. They can eat enormous quantities of food and have difficulty stopping. Beta-endorphin has been well demonstrated in the habits of overeating. Endorphin, our own morphine, makes us feel good. It's a strong neurotransmitter. Like opiates, it kills pain and gives us pleasure.

It has been known for centuries that breathing techniques, such as Lamaze, used during childbirth, can relieve a lot of pain. Chewing food can produce dopamine and endorphin, so eat slowly; it will reduce the appetite. If you eat food quickly, you will not get that effect or benefit.

The hypothalamus, your Wizard of Oz, your metabolic center, controls the appetite through the Carp Center, which turns the appetite off, and your NPY center, which turns appetite on. Lipids from fat and the gremlins in your stomach regulate them. Your survival mechanisms are deep in your hypothalamus; of course, regulating your eating is one of its chief functions.

If an action is needed for your survival, such as reproduction and food consumption, nature has associated pleasure with it. Let's face it—we can overdo both. Food and drug addiction, as well as smoking, seems to travel together in families. The reason is their thought processes generally are probably quite similar. Their habits are quite similar. I recently sat across the table from a very nice large family, spread out along one of those long Japanese tables, so I faced them all directly. From grandchild to grandfather, every single person was seriously overweight. Sad to say, they're going to have a lot of illnesses between them. Psychologically, I wonder, when they look in the mirror, what they really see. Let's face it: we all have some variant of that problem. It's difficult for many of us to face up to reality. I never said life is easy.

Addiction occurs because we are fooling with brain chemistry. An overweight person is likely someone who has been using food to fool with this brain chemistry. It's a malfunction of serotonin metabolism that leads to obesity and overweight. People eat a lot of refined carbohydrates and sugar to improve their mood. I'm familiar with that in my own life. If you have a serotonin malfunction, you will have food cravings. Your body is screaming, "Eat, eat, and eat some more." Your brain is malfunctioning; you are not morally weak. The precursor to serotonin, tryptophan, may not be getting to the brain fast enough. Low-glycemic complex carbohydrates can increase serotonin levels, so avoid refined sugars.

If you are overeating, odds are this is what is happening:

- Your serotonin level is too low.
- You feel depressed.
- You crave sugar products to correct the deficit.
- If you're eating carbs, you increase the insulin level.
- Insulin pushes amino acids into the muscles.
- Tryptophan increases in the blood and enters the brain.
- Serotonin is released, and you feel better, and the appetite is turned down.

Stress releases dynorphin, a powerful appetite stimulant. I know I had a very stressful day on Wednesday—I was up all night doing dangerous surgery, and I did three more routine surgeries the next day without sleep—and I felt I could eat anything all day, and I did. I wonder what my dynorphin level was. We need to have a remedy ready that has been well rehearsed to avoid those situations. Sugar, refined starches, and fat can trigger beta-endorphins and set up a ravenous appetite—EAT, EAT, EAT. Mild stress can release dynorphin and greatly increase the appetite. Relief of stress is rapid after eating, so it gets to be a habit. You must have a remedy ready.

You can see that food is a chemical, and how we think greatly affects our eating habits. It's a war we must face daily. We can solve the problem by developing good habits, and I will teach you what those recommendations will be.

Reversing Type 2 Diabetes

I'm completely convinced that type 2 diabetes can be reversed. I believe it can be done 80 to 90 percent of the time in sixty days. Dr. Franklin House feels he can do it in thirty days. He wrote a famous book, *The 30-Day Miracle*. I've read it a number of times, and I completely agree with it and thank God for finding that book. I've never met an internist who read it. Dr. House has been doing this for twenty-five years and has tremendous experience. Remember that 90 percent of type 2 diabetics become type 1 diabetics.

Dr. Neil Earnhardt feels type 2 diabetes can be reversed as well with a plant-based diet. He's also published a wonderful book describing it. Dr. Joel Fuhrman, the originator of the nutritarian way of eating highly nutrient-dense foods, clearly supports the concept of eliminating type 2 diabetes.

I have read all their books and attended some of their camps and courses. As a matter of fact, I'm leaving again on Friday to attend a one-week seminar with Dr. Joel Fuhrman in San Diego. He is also a big-time tennis player, and I'm really looking forward to this trip. I hope he has practiced a lot, because he's in for a heck of a match. The consensus is the same: the monster of type 2 diabetes can be slain most of the time. Let's get this monkey off your back. Actually, if you ate the way he does, you would be very healthy.

There is now powerful evidence that switching to a healthy way of eating, not dieting, can have a powerful effect on your cells and sugar metabolism. If you have type 2 diabetes, your body doesn't process sugar very well; insulin resistance from fat is the problem. To keep your blood sugar low, you need to avoid processed sugars and fats as much as possible. To avoid all carbohydrates is a mistake; you just need to select them better by using the glycemic index. Limiting your starches like bread, pasta, and rice and eating meat, cheese, white bread, and white rice is a big mistake. A low-carbohydrate diet eventually leads to overeating. The Atkins diet has been a disaster; some of the books I've read called it a fraud.

Because now you're not losing weight on the standard diet recommended by a lot of people, they put you on multiple medications. Many of the medications drop your blood sugar, but now you become hungry and start eating more, which makes the problem worse. Most type 2 diabetics I see are seriously overweight and are on multiple medications to prove the point. They say, "My blood sugar is just fine. Doctor, my diabetes is under control." But you still have diabetes, and you are not taking a look inside your body, where the real problem is. Let's make a plan and get rid of this disease that will give you a lot of trouble in the future. The last twenty years of your life will get very difficult, if you live that long. The most common cause of death in the diabetic is a sudden heart attack without warning.

Besides giving you the normal medications for diabetes, your doctor probably will give you medication for the problems it causes—hypertension, elevated cholesterol and triglycerides—pain medicine for diabetic neuropathy, medicine for losing vision, medications for the effects on your skin, and maybe something for a stroke or heart attack.

Let's look at the study done by Dr. T. Colin Campbell in *The China Study*, a great book to read. He and a group of other doctors under communism studied one billion Chinese people. They looked at their pattern of eating and found a huge correlation to the diseases they developed. The ones eating a plant-based diet had very little illness; the ones eating a fat-based diet had a lot of vascular disease, diabetes, hypertension, and cancer. Disease prevalence varied from region to region depending on how much of these foods the people in each region ate. This study had a lot of medical support. At the end of the study, the researchers could correlate what foods were eaten in different cities based the diseases the residents had. The study gathered a tremendous amount of useful information. Where participants ate a plant-based diet, they had little vascular disease, few heart attacks, few strokes, little dementia, and low cancer rates. That sent us all a huge message. They didn't avoid carbohydrates; they ate more starches than we do. They ate mainly low-glycemic index carbohydrates. They ate rice, grains, vegetables, beans, and some fish. They didn't eat refined foods, foods stripped of their nutrients. They ate brown rice, brown bread, and potatoes with the skin on them and nothing added to them.

In Japan fifteen years ago, only 1 percent of the population was obese, versus 30 percent in the United States. Our fast-food restaurants have moved to Japan, and things are indeed changing. Don't eat in restaurants where the name is the same in every country. Japan had to take on a national initiative to turn the tide of bad eating around. Every employer must measure the waist size of every employee, or they get a huge fine. They even changed the name from obesity to "metabow" after metabolic syndrome, because the people did like the word obese. The Japanese living in Hawaii started eating the American way and are getting sicker. Things even got worse when they moved to California, and now they have American diseases, and even a little bit worse. The reason is they have in their genetic structure, based on evolution, the thrifty gene. If you eat the wrong food, expression of this gene occurs, and you become obese very quickly. Other ethnic groups, such as people from Africa, South America, and Micronesia and the Pima Indians, also have the thrifty genes. They run a very high rate of complications in type 2 diabetes when the gene expresses itself after they eat bad food such as fat, sugar, and salt.

The Asians switched to hamburgers, fried chicken, cheese, and other Western fare, and now they have the same diseases we do. Fat, salt, and sugar are killing them now. Now in Japan, there are fast-food restaurants everywhere, as in the United States. They used to have a 1 percent diabetic rate in Japan, and now it's 12 percent and getting higher. It's the thrifty gene at work. The culprit is the Western diet.

The problem is not carbohydrates, sugar, and starch; the problem is how the body processes them. Carbohydrates do not cause diabetes; it's the fat that causes insulin resistance. Insulin is made by the pancreas, the beta cells located in the islets of Langerhans. A medical student in Germany discovered these islets, which produce insulin, in the 1800s. The insulin made by the pancreas (see illustration) unlocks the door to the cell wall into the cell for energy production. It is supposed to open the gate and let the sugar in, but with insulin resistance, the key to the lock is stuck. It's stuck because fat gums up the receptors; fat in the cell also prevents communication to insulin to open the door.

This is insulin resistance. The key won't work. Our goal is to unlock the door by reducing the fat level in the blood. The fundamental problem in type 2 diabetes is to get the glucose in the cell where it belongs, making energy, or ATP.

A vegan diet, or 80 percent flexitarian or 70 percent nutrient-dense diet (see my book *The Secret of the Non Diet)*, no animal protein, no milk products, no refined foods, plant-based diet, but you can eat all you want. That will do it most of the time.

- Low-glycemic carbohydrates
- Whole grain
- Vegetables
- Beans
- Fruit

A one-point drop in the A1C blood test for the type 2 diabetic can reduce the risk of eye and renal disease tremendously. Actually, it is easy to adjust to this way of eating. Usually in twenty-one days your appetite will change. The tremendous amount of phytochemicals in the food you eat will turn the appetite off. It's a healthy way of eating not only for your blood sugar but also to prevent heart disease, hypertension, dementia, autoimmune diseases, and cancer.

Exercise is a critical part of the plan. Exercise improves insulin resistance tremendously. It will pull the fat out of the cells.

Years ago Dr. Dean Ornish published a great many papers and books about a way of eating to prevent, stop, and reverse vascular disease. His books are great to read. I've read them all a number of times, and some of my patients follow his program. One of my patients was told he needed a heart transplant. Fifteen years later, he is alive and well following the Ornish plan, which is basically what I am teaching. Besides, if you eat the way I recommend, you will be slim and look good and probably add twenty years to your life—and maybe more. Your blood sugar can be corrected very quickly if you follow this type of diet, so you need to contact your doctor and keep adjusting your medications, if you take them. Dr. Franklin House stops oral medications on the first day, to give you an example.

You could be a little bit overweight and the amount of fat in your cells be a little elevated, and you can indeed develop insulin resistance many years before you develop full-blown diabetes. So getting a fasting insulin test should be part of a routine physical. In type 2 diabetes, the little energy factories, the recent research has shown to have few furnaces to burn fat and sugar to make energy. Some research indicates that fat switches off the genes that make your little energy furnaces, the mitochondria, work less.

STRESS AND INSULIN

Stress has tremendous influence on insulin secretion. Insulin controls LPL, which controls fat storage and utilization. That is the key to getting rid of type 2 diabetes. It's the fat that causes inflammation and insulin resistance. Stress plays a big role in that.

Stress is the inability to cope with threats, real or imaginary, to our physical, mental, emotional, and spiritual well-being. That is the best definition of stress in today's society as far as I am concerned. Dr. Hans Selye, the famous researcher who published at least a thousand medical papers on stress, called it the nonspecific response of the body to stress. He did a lot of his studies on animals. He is famous for describing adaptation syndrome.

Stress is everywhere, universal and unending. Stress was here yesterday, it is here today, and it will be here tomorrow, especially in this fast-moving society—with technology, cell phones, e-mails, taxes, and job stress. Multitasking goes on all day, especially in my life, and probably yours.

The World Health Organization predicts by 2020, stress disorders will be the second leading cause of death. Look at my Mind-Body Index on page 28 to give you some idea of the large list of stress illnesses, and it doesn't even list all of them. I've practiced neurology and neurosurgery now for forty-one years, at age thirty-nine. I feel 75 percent of what I'm looking at is a physical presentation of stress in the office. So it is with every other doctor, except many of them do not realize it, unfortunately. Things like fibromyalgia, chronic headaches, neural dermatitis, chronic pain, chronic headaches, and many others are stress illnesses.

We are doing too much to these people. They need stress-reduction techniques and a softer approach. These illnesses can lead to unnecessary tests, injections, CT scans, MRI scans, and operations. Stressed-out people smoke more, drink more, and take more narcotics and illegal drugs. Stress is a megastore of illnesses because it drives up the insulin level, resulting in overeating.

Stress is actually fear. We feel fear because we feel threatened. Stress is felt by a person, but it's just a person's perception of it that affects his or her health. Stress may be real or imaginary. That's why meditation works, because it puts you into the present moment, not the storm of yesterday or the hurricane of tomorrow. When you are living in denial, you are less stressed. We can't tell the real from the imaginary threats. Your brain does not know the difference. Our subconscious mind cannot tell the difference between the saber-toothed tiger and the stress of watching the news on the bad news stations. Yet we have the same physiological response, whether it's real or imaginary. There is no difference between the acute stress of running away from the saber-tooth tiger and the imaginary fears of tomorrow. The biology of stress has been well studied by Dr. Walter Cannon. Around 1910 he studied mainly the acute stress response, which ends quickly and has very little long-term effect on your health if you live through the acute stress. Dr. Hans Selye of Montreal studied chronic stress and long-term stress extensively.

In stress, the frontal lobe sends messages deep into the limbic system of the brain, then to the hypothalamus—the Wizard of Oz, or your brain's brain, the metabolic control center of your brain—which in turn sends cortisone-releasing hormone, CRH, to the pituitary gland, your master gland. The master gland releases adrenocortical trophic hormone, ACTH, which stimulates the adrenal cortex, the gland just above your kidney. The adrenal gland releases glucocorticoid-releasing hormone, cortisol, and catecholamines, epinephrine, and norepinephrine. Your heart rate increases, your respiration increases, your bladder and GI tract stop functioning, your pupils dilate, your skin sweats, your blood pressure goes up, and your metabolic rate increases. You start eating more, especially with chronic stress. A potbelly is a sign of chronic stress. This is the basic stress response carried out by the sympathetic nervous system.

In the face of increased blood sugar and increased blood fats, if the levels spike upward, sugar and fat provide energy for the well-known fight-or-flight response of Dr. Walter Cannon, the acute stress response. You jump higher; you run faster; you lift heavy objects and fight for your life. Remember, the human brain does not distinguish between acute and chronic stress or unreal stress, between minor and life-threatening stress. The response is the same.

We need a lot of energy for the acute stress response. You're running for your life, but the response is the same for the imaginary stressor, which really does not require any significant energy. Now you don't use up the energy from the chronic stress response, which is the most common stress event, and you start gaining weight. That is why stressed-out people have potbellies. They don't use up the energy from the chronic stress response. We don't use up the sugar and fat secreted by the stress response. We eat a lot to relieve stress, because food releases feel-good chemicals, serotonin, dopamine, and endorphins, all opiates that make us feel sleepy and better. It's a vicious cycle. Sometimes the endorphins even produce a ravenous appetite; you just can't stop eating. Believe me, it's happened to me when I've had very stressful days in neurosurgery. Sometimes I can't believe what I've been eating for the last two days. Fortunately, I'm of normal weight because I'm on the straight path most of the time. You get other bad problems of high blood pressure, heart disease, stroke, cancer, dementia, and increased rate of autoimmune diseases, including arthritis. The brain thinks you face the saber-tooth tiger, and appetite goes up, when in reality it was not necessary, because you did not expend the energy you thought you needed. It's all because the chronic stress response is just like the acute stress response, when you indeed need the energy to save your life.

The same steroids brought by the stress response tell the appetite center in your hypothalamus that you're hungry when actually you are not. Once the stress has passed, there's a signal to the hypothalamus to start eating again. It's a totally false signal, and you gain weight. Stress is destructive to the human body.

That is why people eat so much when they are chronically stressed. They will eat the whole bag of potato chips and can't stop. Recently, when I had a very stressful couple of days, I broke my generally good eating habits and ate everything in sight. I couldn't seem to help myself. I had a busy day. I was on call that night, with emergency brain operations and elective surgery the next day. I must have eaten junk food in the hospital for two days. I could not believe what I had done. The body believes we are facing the saber-tooth tiger, that we are about to be killed, when in reality, the threat is not that severe. We eat french fries, bagels, chips, and cakes, foods that cause a rapid rise in fat, salt, and sugar, which is bad for us. It's all about fat. It's difficult to convert whole grains, vegetables, beans, and fruit to fat. It's much more likely to be stored in our muscles or excreted in our bowels. If you eat fat, its stored 97 percent of the time; only 3 percent is lost in metabolism.

Unfortunately, a lot of the fat is stored in the abdomen, not under the skin; it envelops our bowels and pancreas and has great effects on our metabolism. It literally hugs the liver and pancreas, our metabolic centers. Remember, stressed-out people have big bellies. Extra fat was placed there by evolution to be readily available for emergency starvation or metabolism. The increased weight causes insulin levels to rise; you develop insulin resistance; now inflammation arrives, and you have an increased chance of developing cancer, vascular disease, hypertension, and dementia. Your chance of type 2 diabetes increases. Fat is a gland and produces about twenty nasty chemicals, adipokines, and increases a chemical called IGF, a growth-factor chemical, which results in cancer and produces malignant cells. Remember, when Christopher Reeve died, his wife died within a year from cancer with no history of smoking. Stress probably did that. It is well known that following horrible situations like a death or divorce, the rate of cancer increases, as does the rate of sudden death, in the people involved. I have seen it many times in my patients. Stress also is a cause of dementia, because the chemicals in fat affect the neurons of your brain.

Stress management has a part in healing, including the instruction to eliminate fat from your diet as much as possible. Of course, exercise is an important part of the program.

The Brain and Eating: Rudy's Rules

Food is a drug. The chemicals in food break down into serotonin, dopamine, and noradrenaline, the feel-good chemicals. Now you feel great, but you're killing yourself with all the sugars and processed foods. You have to make a decision to eat right and reduce your sugar craving. I suggest before every meal, you apply Rudy's Rules: take a minute and visualize your intention. To remember your goal, visualize yourself as a healthy person—no diabetes, no young-age blindness, stroke, or sudden heart attack. Take that minute before every meal. You've made your decision; you have a plan; now send a message through visualization to your subconscious mind: "I have made up my mind to change. I want to live a healthy life."

Remember the diet of your ancestors: nuts, berries, vegetables, and low-fat meat—not the mad, sad, toxic diet of today. There has not been enough time in terms of evolution to change our bodies; that's why we're getting sick. Remember, fat causes insulin resistance. The fat interferes with the ability of insulin to transport sugar into the cell for metabolism. You need sugar for energy. High insulin in the blood causes fat deposits and arteriosclerosis—just what you don't want.

Eating healthy low-glycemic-index carbohydrates is a step in the right direction. Low-glycemic-index carbohydrates do not cause diabetes. We're talking about carbohydrates with fiber in them. A way of eating that involves 20 percent protein, 20 percent low saturated fat, and 60 percent low-glycemic-index carbohydrates is an excellent way of eating. In my book *The Secret of a Non Diet* is a list of high-fiber, low-glycemic-index, and highly nutrient-dense foods. Don't eat a high-protein diet. Animal protein has a lot of fat and cholesterol. Fatty triglycerides in the blood cause fat storage in the cells and can increase cell size a thousand times. Fat in the cells prevents insulin receptors from working and shuts down the transportation system. Your body cells, seventy trillion of them, are your minibrains. Cell metabolism is very complex.

Fat is the grease in the cell that locks up the insulin receptors, which causes type 2 diabetes. It locks the door from the outside and inside. If you're slightly overweight, you could still have the beginning of insulin resistance. Get a serum insulin test, a very accurate test that can anticipate type 2 diabetes.

Animal protein is very dangerous. It is high in fats and cholesterol, which leads to disease and inflammation. Animal protein is very hard on the kidneys and liver. There is plenty of protein in plants. Diabetes is the most common cause of kidney disease and renal transplants.

Fiber is your friend and filter. It prevents absorption of many fats. That is why a nutrient-dense diet with a lot of fiber is great for avoiding obesity and diabetes. Fiber prevents metabolism of 40 percent of the low-glycemic-index foods. If you eat a hundred calories of fat, 97 percent will sit on your abdomen or buttocks within four hours. Only 3 percent will be metabolized. If you eat a low-glycemic-index carbohydrate, 40 percent will be metabolized, so eat a great deal more of that type of food. Meat and cheeses have no fiber. Low-fiber diets are not healthy.

Macronutrients—fat, carbohydrates, and protein—are the basic food energy chemicals. The micronutrients are sixteen minerals, fourteen vitamins, and twenty thousand phytochemicals. They are the enzymes and coenzymes that regulate your metabolism and have no caloric value. One gram of fat has nine calories; one gram of protein has four calories. You can see the problem of fat; it has a lot more calories per gram.

What's Your Situation: The Scoreboard

Find out your body mass index. If it's over thirty, you're overweight. If it's over thirty-five, you're obese. If it's over forty, it is called morbid obesity. Don't panic; this can be stopped, prevented, and reversed. Within thirty to sixty days, a short period of time, I will help you. Sometimes waist measurements are used, but frankly this is not as good as my BMI tables, which are readily available for adults and children.

You might also look at a website called bluezones.com. It asks you about thirty-three questions. Based on your habits, it will give you an estimate of your biological age, not chronological. It may motivate you into action. Focus on your health; how you think is everything. If you keep doing what you're doing, don't expect different results.

Ways of Eating

- Vegetarians don't eat meat. Vegetarians live ten years longer than most of us.
- Vegans don't eat meat or dairy products—an excellent way of eating.
- Flexitarian—that's Rudy's way of eating—80 percent vegan, 20 percent fish.
- Nutritarian—highly nutrient-dense foods, some low-fat meat.

What Does "Nutrient Dense" Mean?

Nutrient-dense foods are foods that have not been stripped of their minerals, vitamins, and phytochemicals, including fresh vegetables, beans, and fruits and low-glycemic-index complex carbohydrates and grains. Calorie-dense foods that have been stripped of the vitamins, minerals, and phytochemicals are, in essence, processed foods such as doughnuts, cookies, candies, white bread, and white rice. Whole grains, leafy greens, orange and yellow fruits and vegetables, citrus fruits, peppers, broccoli, raw nuts, and seeds are all nutrient-dense foods.

I also recommend you take a supplement of multivitamins and ground flaxseed to get omega-3. Make vegetables the foundation of your meals. Put a sign on your refrigerator that says: If hunger is not what you have, food is not what you need. Don't eat anything you're not willing to kill.

A pound of vegetables, beans, and legumes has only a hundred calories and lots of volume. Serve soybeans and edamame several times a week. They are very healthy, and they taste good. Soybean products are an excellent source of protein and phytochemicals.

Fruits are nature's perfect food. Our closest primate relatives eat only fruit. Fruits have formal fiber, vitamins, minerals, phytochemicals, and antioxidants. You should have at least two or three servings per day.

You only need about 35 to 55 grams of protein. We eat about 140 grams daily with a lot of fat and cholesterol. Proteins are the building blocks for enzymes, neurotransmitters, neuropeptides, and muscle. There's plenty of protein in plants; you don't need to eat animal protein. The American and

Canadian Dietetic Association states that a vegetarian diet is healthy for adults and children. If you are on a high-protein diet, you're much more likely to have osteoporosis.

You should need only about 20 percent of fat in your diet. You need some fat, but it needs to be good fat that comes from essential fatty acids, the twenty-carbon omega-3 fatty acids. You should get them from nuts, fish, or flaxseed. The omega-3s lead to good eicosanoids, the Intel chips of your body, and are very important. Fat builds walls of our cells, it is part of all hormones and the precursor of good and bad eicosanoids, and you do use some fat for energy. Fats can be polyunsaturated, saturated, trans, monounsaturated, omega-3, and omega-6, good and bad. The more hydrogen ions fat has, the more saturated it becomes.

Trans fats are from plant oils that have had a hydrogen atom added and are now solid at room temperature. When they start to decay, they do a lot of damage to your body. Omega-3 and omega-6 should be in a one-to-one relationship in your diet. Most Americans have a ratio of fifteen to one, omega-6 to omega-3, a very dangerous situation. Some examples of foods that contain trans fats are french fries, doughnuts, cookies, and so on. All plant oils are 100 percent fat. Olive oil is not a health food, but a tablespoonful is certainly reasonable.

A plant-based diet is full of antioxidants. Because of vitamins, minerals, and phytochemicals, free radicals are caused by food and are part of metabolism. Free radicals cause accelerated aging and dementia. The larger share of antioxidants come from plants—God's food. Artificial foods are bad because of free radicals. Processing strips food of vitamins, minerals, and phytochemicals. White flour is very unhealthy. Sugar is a disaster; we eat approximately 150 pounds yearly. Sugar is the devil's food. It is the biggest cause of heart attacks and strokes. Increased sugar levels in the blood lead to increased body fat and arteriosclerosis. Saturated fats and sugar are a disaster; read the labels for fat and sugar content. Healthy carbohydrates contain fiber. There are plenty of carbohydrates in plants. Fiber is the undigested compounds of plant cell walls. Fiber has tremendous benefits for diabetes. Fiber delays emptying of the stomach and slows absorption of food. Fiber reduces the absorption of fats, sugars, LDL, and cholesterol.

Motivating Change

As a physician, I consider myself to be a teacher; after all, that is what the word "physician" means. So I have a built-in desire to make people well. Frankly, I like to be called Dr. Wellness. The mayor of our city called me that at a recent meeting. And I am proud of that. Being a physician, of course, I see patients every day who need wellness teaching. They wouldn't come to see me if they had no problems. But how do you facilitate change? How do you motivate someone toward wellness? I do take the time, maybe even thirty minutes, to educate the patient toward wellness. It's a noble desire to change someone; it's actually my job. We may certainly differ in what the right path is. Motivation is an interpersonal process—an interaction between two people. Motivation for change cannot only be influenced by us but, in a very real sense, arises from an interpersonal context. We may assume that the person is already motivated for change when he comes to see us, but most of the time that is not true. Many want a quick fix, a pill, a procedure, or maybe even an operation, which may not be needed. I see that all the time. Exploring and enhancing motivation for change is a necessary task for us and our physician, if we plan to get well. Many times, the person you're trying to change, including yourself, is ambivalent about the need for it. The patient should be voicing the arguments for change, or you yourself may express these opinions and feel the need for it. But that is not always the case. If I or the patient is voicing arguments against change, I have to be very careful as to what I say, or I will never convince him or her to do it. Both parties often leave the interaction dissatisfied, each blaming the other, and very little positive change occurs. I have had it happen to me more than once, trying to convince a patient to follow a certain course of wellness instead of having injections or operations or using narcotics for his or her nonspecific pain. Motivational interviewing is more like dancing rather than struggling against each other. You have to move together smoothly; otherwise nothing will happen. Motivating change needs imagination. You have to develop and point out discrepancies in the other person's interpretation of his or her present state of health, between how he or she thinks and what actual reality is. You may think you look good being overweight, but you're not looking at what's going to occur in the future. You're not looking at what is going on inside your body: diabetes, arthritis, heart disease, and so on. The discrepancy is generally between the present status and a desired goal of good health. The difference is between what is happening and how we would like things to be—to be healthy, look good, and live a long life. The larger the discrepancy, the greater the importance of change. Because it involves perception, however, discrepancy is more complex than just noticing the difference between what is and what should be. One's behavior can come into conflict with a deeply held value without they're being a change in either. I've heard it many times: "Although I have heart disease and diabetes, I can't give up eating meat." This happens particularly when there is a change not in the behavior but in the perceived meaning of the behavior. When a behavior comes into conflict with a deeply held value, it is usually the behavior that changes. So it is very important to know what the deeply held values are. That might motivate us to change. For example, a person might decide to stop smoking so his or her children don't become sick. Some people are ambivalent about taking the first step toward change. As the discrepancy increases, ambivalence first intensifies; then if the discrepancy continues to grow, ambivalence can be resolved in the direction of change. Ambivalence is not really an obstacle to change; it is what makes change possible. So the challenge is to first to identify and then resolve ambivalence by developing discrepancy between the actual present situation and the desired future. It can be very difficult.

When I'm speaking to patients to change them in a thirty-minute interview, a number of them completely agree while in front of me and even express a desire to change; the husband and wife may both agree, but nothing happens. Others go to my wellness center and buy my books and DVDs and continue their education to change. Follow-up appointments are very important so that I can remotivate patients. I encourage them to attend my lectures, which are free, for further education. Of course, attending the lectures is a sign of motivation and many times does induce change. Change is facilitated by communicating in a way that elicits a person's own reasons for an advantage of change. I examined a patient like that yesterday and took full advantage of his pointing out the discrepancy in his behaviors. He was killing himself from type 2 diabetes. I pointed out to him the disadvantages of the status quo. I pointed out to him the advantages of change. I prayed for his optimism to change, that he could get the job done, and he expressed an intention to change. I tried to get him to commit to change in front of his wife. To get someone else involved with the commitment increases the chances of that actually happening.

Mind, Body, Spirit

Knowledge of the connection of mind, body, and spirit can be very motivating. Our body has a doctor living in it. It needs to be awakened; it knows how to get us well. There's a connection of the mind with the body and the body with the mind. Dr. Candice Pert wrote a famous book called *Molecules of Emotion*. It explains the effects of your brain through neuropeptides (three hundred of them), hormones, and neurotransmitters in your sixty trillion body cells. The sixty trillion body cells speak back to your body and brain with your eicosanoids, the Intel chips of your body made by every cell of your body. So how you think is everything. Your thought process leads the way. No matter what your health problem is, how you think can have tremendous effects on these diseases and your well-being. Many can be cured by the proper practice of wellness, diet, exercise, and positive thinking. Many patients are not motivated to get better, some due to lack of knowledge of the mind-body connection, some due to the healthcare provider, who has no idea of the mind-body connection. This is, unfortunately, quite common. I know a number of cancer specialists who have no understanding whatsoever of the mind-body connection. The work of Dr. Carl Simonton and Dr. La Shan has proven the benefits of mind-body techniques in the treatment of cancer. Studies have shown cancer patients can live twice as long if they practice mind-body techniques; the spontaneous cure rate increases. The scientific proof goes back centuries. The will to live has a commanding influence on motivation. Patients want their bodies fixed, but some don't want to be part of the team.

What Is Holistic Medicine?

- You look at the physical aspect of the disease.
- You look at the physiology of the disease.
- You look to the spiritual aspect of the patient.
- The patient must participate in the belief of his or her recovery.
- The love of the family is important.
- A placebo doctor needs to be part of the team, as well as the patient.

What's Going On in Your Life?

Stress is a cause of numerous illnesses. I made a list of the illnesses caused by stress and put them in the Mind-Body Index, a name I copyrighted, just like a body mass index. I did that so that the public and the medical providers would pay more attention to illness caused by stress. We really don't find anything on any test. Yet a lot of operations on these patients are done unnecessarily, because they don't understand the concept of mind-body illness. Illness is the perception of being unwell. A partial list all of these illnesses are illustrated here—these illnesses can plague a patient, who can spend a lifetime with them. Once a person has been educated to believe his or her illness is due to stress and the symptoms are real, then the healing can begin. Education is the motivation factor in my experience. It may take some work. Some patients and families are just incredulous when I tell them it's a stress problem and nothing life threatening is going on. They have been so fixated on an MRI report and believed their body was falling apart, when it's only the process of aging and nothing unusual. The overreliance on CT scans, MRIs, and angiograms is a serious problem, leading to a lot of unnecessary medical care. The interpretation of these studies and their relationship to the patient's symptoms is the critical factor. A lot of it depends whether you going to a placebo or a nocebo healthcare provider. Read my chapter on placebo for more details. A placebo doctor educates the patient with some material to read and recommends DVDs, CDs, and meditation, which can motivate the patient to wellness. It may take a few visits to get the job done, but that is the job of the family physician to start. If the family physician is not a motivator or a placebo doctor, it's a real problem, because 50 to 75 percent of the patients need that. You can take the stress test associated with my Mind-Body Index to judge the probability of you having or developing a mind-body disease. The point is, if you can see the connection, if you have one of these mind-body illnesses, you can be cured. You can avoid a lot of unnecessary procedures by reading my book *Welcome to Your Mind-Body*. It explains the mind-body connection in detail. It can save you a lot of pain, unnecessary procedures, and a lot of money. If you don't have a mind-body disease, I guarantee you, your friends or relatives have one, and maybe they have them all, as I've seen in some of my patients. My educating them has helped a great deal.

A Sense of Purpose

How can we continue doing the same thing and expect a different outcome? We all want a better life, better health, financial gains, determination to beat that serious illness, and a whole host of other things that we anticipate will give us that sense of purpose we so desire. How can we accomplish these huge goals? What will get us progressing in the right direction? As a wellness doctor and lecturer, I give both patients and audiences the education and the scientific background to stimulate change by teaching the wellness aspect of illness and disease. But is that really enough to get the job done? How motivating am I? Do my words lead to short-term or long-term changes in my listeners? I've certainly seen changes in my patients, some short term and others long term, and yet I suspect some others do not change at all. I practice what I preach, and I presume that to be motivating. And so I aim for long-term changes in my patients. Correlation is used to urge interaction, but it may be short term. What you need is change that endures. You must be proactive if you plan to change your life. Changes need to be started immediately, or the commitment will leave you. Consistency in what you are doing can leave quickly as feelings interfere. Now you have another failed attempt, and you feel discouraged. A shaky commitment can get in the way of purposeful motivation. Creating a sense of purpose for your life and doing something to duplicate that is more likely to result in a permanent change and your accomplishing your goal. When you set out to create and accomplish, while stimulated by this sense of purpose, you are most likely to cause these long-term changes within yourself. Motivation solves short-term problems, but for long-term results, you must find the root of your sense of purpose and renovate it. When we are fearful, we go for quick fixes. Drugs, cigarettes, and food are all chemicals that affect the mind for a quick fix. And of course that only leads to more problems—poor health, family conflict, job loss. The list goes on and on. If you develop a sense of purpose in life, you are most likely to reach your long-term goal, and your subconscious mind will help you to get there. The famous cancer psychotherapist Dr. Lawrence LeShan found during forty-five years of treating cancer patients that if he could find or discover a purpose in life for his cancer patient, he could double his or her lifespan and increase the likelihood of a spontaneous cure of the cancer. A sense of purpose stimulates activity in the immune system, improving both longevity and cure rate. Now sit down with a pencil and paper, and write down what you are trying to accomplish, whether it be weight loss, transforming your appearance, improving family relations, a career change, or getting rid of bad habits such as smoking and/or drinking. If you establish a sense of purpose to improve yourself, it is much more likely you will reach your goal and make it happen. For example, although I am in my early seventies, I have created a sense of purpose by planning to be the national eighty-and-over tennis champ. I am already training for it. I take a tennis lesson once a week from the best player in town, do yoga and weight training three days a week, and play tennis at night on a regular basis. It has given me a reason to get out of bed, and I have a sense of great purpose. This is what motivates me. Additionally, I am writing books, creating DVDs, giving a great number of lectures on wellness, and practicing neurosurgery full-time. At seventy-three, I have developed a sense of purpose that is very motivating. I wake early at five o'clock and start my day reading, writing, working out, and practicing my saxophone. By nine o'clock, I take a pause at Starbucks to meet friends and get ready for the day's work. I can't say it enough: I feel a great sense of purpose in helping others get well. I hope you can find your purpose in life. It will motivate you to get the job done. Look for a sense of purpose, like getting in shape.

For example, type II diabetes is curable in thirty days by eating the right foods. Or improve the relationships within your family. If you have self-induced physical problems, eliminate them. Think of this—if you die, it is your family that will suffer. You need to find your song, the one that makes you move permanently in the direction of your goals and gives vision to your life. We all have a unique song to sing no matter what the circumstance. Find your unique individual music and make it positive! It will improve your self-image, and it will be a call to action. All people have a natural way of relating and creating, and when you find yours, you will fulfill your dreams. You need to take control of your own life; no one will do it for you. "I just can't do it" are not acceptable words. Visualize a life you would like to live, and work toward it every day, even if you are only making small changes. The changes will stimulate your immune system and your subconscious mind, and visualizing it will make it much more likely to happen. We can keep on doing the same things and expect different results, but that is just insanity. When you have discovered your purpose, immediately begin to create momentum. Write down your purpose or goal frequently, and then do something daily to work toward this goal with some positive action. Set a three-month, six-month, and one-year goal, and have a little celebration when you achieve these goals. Helping others may be the most motivating thing you can do; it sure works for me. Spirituality and religion create purpose for many people. Senseful purpose is the food on which our souls can thrive. Your age does not matter—use me as an example. We all need something to strive toward, so we can design our own inspiration. This will be different for different people. The secret to living is to create a meaningful purpose. The first step to creating any change is to decide what you want, not what you don't want. That is what will create a purpose in your life. Twenty percent of change is to know how to create it; and if you have opposition to change, you need to know why you're doing it. Dr. Rick Warren, the famous evangelist, affirms that purpose is not a list of goals. Goals are temporary; purposes are eternal. It is a statement that points the direction of your life. He would say that if you tie your direction to your spiritual leader, whether that be God, Mohammed, or Jesus, it is much more likely to happen. Writing down your purposes forces you to think specifically about the path of your life, and knowing which way you are headed will keep you on solid ground. An intelligent person knows the direction he or she is going, but a fool starts going off in many different directions. Find out what your purpose is, and start working on it today.

SELF-DISCIPLINE AND ENTHUSIASM

Enthusiasm exaggerates the importance of things and overlooks the deficiencies. Self-discipline motivates you into a realistic direction. Enthusiasm can be wasted energy, and it may not be good. Then again, it does have some value. Self-discipline is taking control of your thoughts, habits, and emotions. Self-discipline must be done daily. You never master it completely, but it becomes easier with practice. You watch what you eat daily, thoughtfully, and eventually it will be a habit, and you won't have to think about it every time you take a bite. The same with exercise then, daily or multiple times per week. After about six weeks, it is just a habit, thoughtless, and is something you just do, like being nice to people on a regular basis. Complete dedication is the extreme of self-discipline; highly successful people exhibit this trait. If you want a huge change in your health habits, you must have self-discipline and dedicate yourself to get the job done. Small changes are motivating. We all can do that; it does not take a special person. You just have to make up your mind to do it. You must motivate yourself to make the sacrifices. Just think: you could get rid of type II diabetes in thirty to sixty days. What a triumph. Sometimes you need to have self-discipline, dedication, sacrifice, a coordinated plan, and maybe a few sleepless nights to turn a bad habit around. The price needs to be paid. You can if you think you can. The common denominator of success to wellness over another person who doesn't achieve it lies in the fact that you have good habits to do it and the failing person doesn't. The failing person will be obese and get diabetes, heart attacks, and strokes at a younger age, as well as an increased chance of cancer. So the path to wellness is important. Any resolution or decision you make has no value and is worth nothing until you make a habit of wellness and stick to it. You have to make the change every day, keep it every day, and if you miss one day, you have to go back and start all over. The kind of determination and commitment required is a good dose of self-discipline and persistence. Anyone can do it if they want to. The ultimate competition exists within us. What you do will eventually be your habits, and your habits will be your character. Enthusiasm can be overdone. It's self-discipline that gets the job done and is very motivating.

Positive Thinking

It is very difficult to improve your life if you think negatively. It is much easier to motivate yourself if you start your day with a positive attitude. Your brain speaks to your seventy trillion body cells with neuropeptides (three hundred of them), hormones, and neurotransmitters. Your seventy trillion cells in turns speak to your brain. Mind-body, body-mind. So how you think has a tremendous effect on how you feel and what you might do. The king of writing about positive thinking is Dr. Norman Vincent Peale. I recommend you read his books. I met one of his assistant ministers a few years ago; he was elderly and said he had all of Dr. Peale books. He said he would never read them again and gave them to me as a present. Many of them were autographed by Dr. Norman Vincent Peale and his lovely wife, Ruth. I am forever grateful. I have read them all about three times. Dr. Peale says, "Positive thinkers get positive results." Clearly, he recommends tying your life to spirituality to create life-changing activity. He suggests a number of basic principles that will motivate your life to your goals, and especially wellness. There is a deep tendency in human nature to become precisely what we imagine or picture ourselves to be. It decides where our life is heading. Negative thinking is a self-destructive process. He who constantly sends out negative thoughts activates the world negatively. That is the law of attraction, which has been widely written about also. Thoughts that are alike attract each other. Negative thoughts result in negative results. If your thinking does not change, don't expect a different result. Our thoughts, through neuropeptides, hormones, and neurotransmitters, affect the immune system and can kill or heal us. Our thought process affects the Intel chips of our body, the eicosanoids, and the super hormones. Seventy trillion body cells are greatly affected by our eicosanoids, the communicators. Our white cells make all the neuropeptides our brain makes. Brain-body, body-brain. The positive thinker sends out positive thoughts with images of hope, optimism and creativity. The greatest discovery of our generation is that human beings can alter their lives by altering their attitudes of the mind. Every problem contains the seeds of its own solution. A positive thinker doesn't react emotionally when in difficulty. The positive thinker is aware that only being cool, with strong mental control, will produce rational sound solutions. Calm thoughts produce results. The negative principle negates. You will not motivate wellness. The positive concept will motivate you to change. The positive principle goes for victory. Inspiration and motivation are like nutrition; you have to keep taking daily and in good amount. Remember, there's more strength and power in the individual and his or her ability to change toward wellness. We use only 10 percent of our abilities on a regular basis; our real potential is huge. Write on a card what you intend to be in life; keep the card for constant reference, and embed that goal deeply in your mind for a period of years. You will become what you said you would like to achieve. Motivation is like nutrition. You must take it daily. Remember, you're doing only about 10 percent of what you could do. Life has an "if" at the center; take control of that. There is magic in believing in yourself. Use imaging and visualization; see your future clearly—what your wellness goals are, what you would like to get rid of in your body, physical and mental fitness—see it. Make a commitment to the principle of wellness. You can if you think you can. Forget the word "impossible." Even if you have only a little faith like a grain of mustard seed, "Nothing shall be impossible unto you" (the Bible). Some people are happier being defeated—a sick mental attitude. Don't be paralyzed in your head. Rebuild your motivation; become a specialist in the possible; take the "I'm" out of impossible. Remember, faith is the most powerful of all forces. Nothing can get you down if you have faith. Know for sure there is a giant within you. Then release the giant "YOU." Don't get down. If you think you failed, just recommit and don't look back. The secret of genius is to carry the spirit of the child into old age. The ability to meet adversity—in failure, sorrow and misfortune—with a smile and renewed enthusiasm for the future is really the secret of life. We're all going to have troubles sometimes. To keep going with enthusiasm at a high level is one of the most exciting things about the positive principle. Failure is only an incident of a successful life. It happens. Get up and develop a new motivational strategy, image and visualize it, and get to work. Keep enthusiasm going in your life now and forever. The words "old age" or "aging" are not in my language. "When are you going to retire, Doctor?" is a question that really makes me mad. "What are you going to do next, Doctor? When is your next book coming out? When are you playing the next tennis tournament?" are better questions. If you fear inferiority, endure it no longer. Every night free your mind of negative thoughts, just as you empty your pockets. Keep positive, and nothing will ever be too much for you. Faith and spirituality are the enemies of fear and are motivating. Form a mental picture or image of the goal you wish to achieve. Dr. Peale would pray, visualize, energize, and actualize. This procedure is a powerful force. It's a creativity principle. Goals are dreams with deadlines. You never know what you can do until you really try—really try. Trying is a continuous process that needs to be sustained at a high level if it is to achieve its goal. Use the power of imagination, creative imaging and visualization, the language of your subconscious mind. Picture your goal, and run to it with daily affirmations and positive statements. Cool it; don't panic. Last year the stock market almost crashed; I was frozen at the computer. I do my own trading. Think hard. Get help. Get motivated. Sitting there panicking, doing nothing, won't do. The human mind cannot function at its best when it is overheated. Think objectively, not emotionally. Learn to meditate to calm yourself. Get Rudy's prescription for stress reduction from our website, www.kachmannmindbody.com. Never vaguely and indecisively fool around with a difficulty; take a hold and handle it. Get in contact with the energy of the universe. The Chinese way of thinking embraces the Tao, the universal energy, a life-force concept. The truth is we can constantly be in a re-creative process through which the power for life-force is ever giving us renewed vitality. Life is energy. Dr. Peale carried on an extremely active schedule of writing, speaking, editing, public speaking, and administration. He kept his own energy and vitality going by constant affirmations of the life-force, visualizing it as continuously flowing through his mind. He became tired, but a night's sleep always cured things. Let's face it—he had a highly purposeful life, and that is very motivating. Don't drag through life. A multitude of people drag through life in a dreary sort of way, having little or no zest. They may have very little wrong with them, but life is not very invigorating for them. When a person of this type has a real energizing and vital experience, he is astounded by the new quality of his life. Thomas Edison said, "If we did all the things that we are capable of, we would literally astound ourselves." Empty the mind of all unhealthy thoughts; replace them with creativity. Visualize a life-force operating within you, connecting you and refreshing your body, mind, and spirit. Affirm it daily with positive statements. Get in harmony with the basic rhythm of life. Connect all your activities to the positive principle. Remember, fear and negativity can destroy; faith and positive thinking can create and develop. Reprogram your thinking, and become a practitioner of the positive principle. Then miracles will start to happen. The best is yet to be. Live your life, and forget your age. It's a spiritual experience that really changes things, the in-depth type that brings you to life and keeps your life every day all the way. Develop strong mental shields to ward off the bombardment of negatives. Keep contact with spiritual retreat of power, and you will always and forever keep the positive principle going. Think future. I'd like to live to be a hundred years old and be of sound mind. To achieve that, you will need to live a life of wellness, physically and mentally. Ninety percent of type 2 diabetics become type I diabetics.

Don't Sit Still: Move

We teach our children to sit still. Certainly, there are times when this is necessary, or at least we think so, such as in school and church and so on. We obsessed about it years ago. We should do more "walking" lectures in school and maybe stand up for at least ten minutes per hour, have some corporate board meetings where it's okay to stand the whole or part of the time. It could become a habit or nothing unusual to do this. Certainly, it would take some adjusting. Imagine it; visualize it—a nation of movers. How much AOL did you do today?

It has been scientifically proven that we have sitting and standing enzymes in our body that are activated by light activity and not by running a marathon, for example. Yes, mild to moderate physical activity turns enzymes on or off and affects our metabolism.

Stand-up desks, or SUDs, and treadmills with computers are starting to appear in offices. I visited a marketing firm the other day, and they had ten treadmill computers and half a dozen stand-up desks. I shook the hand of their forward-thinking boss. Besides, he was sponsoring lunch-and-learns about health, which I have spoken at. What a great place to work.

Offices are mainly in cubicles spaces now, but they do have some increased socialization, which could result in better health habits. When we look at each other more, we can meet workout buddies, we can educate each other, we can increase our AOL by moving around the office every chance we get. There are opportunities there.

These huge office complexes could essentially be turned into gyms, filled with AOL, especially in the bigger cities, which generally are better at health-promotion ideas. Besides, it is easier to walk down the sidewalks during lunch hours. Some people are walking, standing, using computer treadmills and light weights at their desk, and using every opportunity they can. Lunch breaks can involve a lot of movement. A relative of mine walks through the Millennium Park in Chicago every lunch hour, lucky guy. Remember, if you increase your calorie burn by two hundred calories a day, that means a twenty-pound weight loss in a year. Wow!

Especially since we have cell phones and iPads, we can stand up and walk with them while we're using them. In essence, you are exercising with them or increasing your AOL. I encourage you to keep track of your steps and try to reach at least ten thousand a day. A Fitbit will give you the number. We find tethered you from the cords and wireless, so take advantage of it to get on the move. Use the stairs, not the elevator. Count the hours you're standing. You may be surprised—hopefully, pleasantly. By moving, bouncing, fiddling, walking, and running, you can rest in the hereafter. Aim for 105 years of age; you have a high chance of doing that. Visualize it.

Sitting atrophies your muscles, destroys your posture, and turns you into a hunchback. Our bodies are not designed to sit. That's the reason our enzymes turn off when we don't move. Frankly, it's sitting that makes us fat. Play sports, sports that you love, watching sports is for for others. The American Medical Association through one of its officials said that sitting excessively is nothing short of deadly. We knew that already. So it's not just sugar the booger, it's too much sitting too.

An article in *Time* magazine said that "sitting is sabotaging your health." It recommended "deskersize." Turn your desk into a gym. Let's face it: if you could do your AOL at work, that would make your life a lot easier. It's easier, it's cheaper, and it will make you healthy. It also will be a great example for your fellow workers and your children. Varidesk is a good website for selection of treadmill desks, stand-up desks, and a lot of other technology and apparatuses that can be used in the office or at work.

If your employer does not wish to pick up the cost, then consider buying it yourself. Remember, good health is worth $1 million or more, especially when you don't have it.

As a *New York Times* article said in October, "The idea that a person should not move seems to have taken a hike"! The *New York Times* "Style" section in October had a great selection of fashionable SUDs. Furniture has been invented for schools, and a few have made them available to the children. How forward-looking that is. We could train children in school how to increase their movement throughout their life, in school as well as at home. We would have a much healthier nation.

Fortunately, times are changing, and workplaces are developing more and more "move and shake activities"—at work this might help turn this epidemic of overweight, obesity, and their horrible complications around. The results could be fantastic. Eat less sugar and increase your AOL, eat 70–80 percent nutrient-dense foods, and you can live to be one hundred. It's not that hard.

Technology helped create the problem, but technology can also solve it!

I Was Blind, but Now I See

I was at a large healthcare fair last Saturday and Sunday. A few people walking by spoke to me, knowing that I teach wellness. Actually, I was going to give a lecture on sitting disease a little bit later there. I walked around, and not being judgmental but looking at the health aspects of people, after all that was the purpose of this fair, I would say 90 percent of the people were overweight. Probably 90 percent of them were prediabetic and not aware of it. Fortunately, or unfortunately for my eyes, I could guess the person's blood sugar most of the time, unless he or she just ate a big meal. Frankly, if I knew what they ate, I could probably be pretty accurate again. What concerned me was, of course, the majority probably were undiagnosed and on the road to type 2 diabetes.

Even with gentle encouragement, many refuse to have their blood tested. We live in denial a great deal. Then again, many don't know the many complications of diabetes, or they just don't want to know. Frankly, if they really knew the future, they would be more likely to get tested. Then again, many of them have relatives with advanced chronic disease.

I was able to talk a number of them into getting blood tests, many found out the next day from the labs that 93 percent were abnormal. They were lost, but now they are found. Hopefully, they will act on it. I also encouraged them to attend my free monthly lecture on preventing, stopping, and reversing diabetes in thirty days at the Lutheran Hospital in Fort Wayne, Indiana. Interestingly enough, I donated the three-hundred-seat auditorium to the hospital about thirty-five years ago so the doctors would take advantage of it and teach patients, but I'm the main doctor using it.

What would make people refuse the test? It was free. They were probably living in denial or delusion or both. Do they just not want to know? Is there a lack of knowledge? Are they afraid of the dark?

When I feel stressed, not thinking of it certainly helps. I'll worry about tomorrow. It's too scary to some people to discuss the reality of it. Then again, prevention, stopping disease, and even reversing it can be a very exhilarating trip. Our lives are too complex already, so why face another problem? Who knows for sure?

As already mentioned get your child tested yearly, starting at birth. Now you're living in reality, and to prevent illness of your child in the future will be great deal brighter. No unannounced sudden death from heart disease at age thirty. Believe me, I've seen it more than once.

Incidentally, some people are of normal weight yet are on the prediabetic path, so blood testing is king here. Asians especially can be thin and still have prediabetes or diabetes of an advanced nature. We can look great but our blood work still be very abnormal. You are what your blood work is. If your blood work is normal, you won't have to worry about your health as much, especially if you are exercising a little bit. So let's participate in our healthcare.

Dr. Jeffrey S. Bland wrote a great book called *The Disease Delusion*, endorsed by Dr. Mark Hyman. They are singing the same tune, which I agree with, and I recommend you read it. Dr. Mark Hyman's website has on it *How to Speak to Your Doctor*. I encourage you to read it. It can give you the reasons and what a test to get for to catch you as early as possible and apostle path to diabetes. I highly recommend getting the test that he writes about.

Culture of Wellness Circle

Let's bring it full circle about being well psychologically, physically, and emotionally, not just about nutrition or the amount of exercise, although they play a huge part.

I put together the wellness wheel of eight basic recommendations on what it takes to be well. It is based on my more than fifty years of being a doctor, publishing many CDs, DVDs, and over twenty books and running two TV shows as well as one radio show on wellness. Obviously, I'm still learning every day, but I do have a lot of experience, and I practice what I preach. I'm celebrating the forty-first anniversary of my thirty-ninth birthday next April 25 and have no obvious health problem. I exercise at least two hours a day.

I spend a lot of time with my patients, although as a neurosurgeon, teaching them to get well without injections, medications, or surgery. Generally, I think the patients liked it, but I'm not sure the hospital did, or even my partners. I was spending a lot of time with the patients. My opening statement generally was, "What's going on in your life" Unless you fell out of airplane or just got shot.

Self-responsibility and participating in your healthcare are most important. I don't accept just-script to the ill. Your provider needs to talk to you at every visit and review some things you might do to improve your health. Not just prescriptions, pills, injections, and surgery right off the bat, unless it's an emergency.

Number two is nutrition, which plays a huge part in your health. What are you eating? America has a 70–80 percent overweight population, which leads to the majority of the chronic diseases we're looking at. Dr. David Katz, for thirty-five years the biggest public health official in the nation, on the cover of his book *Disease-Proof* says that 93 percent of diabetes, 80 percent of vascular disease, and 60 percent of cancer can be totally avoided by watching how you use your fingers, what you put on your fork, and how you use your feet. Wow. This speaks of prevention and is represented very well on the wellness wheel.

Dr. Joel Fuhrman is a nationally known physician whom you may have seen on PBS, he has written the best-selling books *Eat to Live* and *End of Diabetes*, for example. He says health equals nutrients/calories represent great health. I agree with that. It is the symphony, mosaic, rainbow, and music of interaction of vitamins, minerals, and phytochemicals that lead to good health.

As already mentioned earlier in this book, an easier way to accomplish this is to read the chapter on sitting disease. The combination of AOL, taking advantage of the thermic effect of food, which causes great calorie burn and prevents, stops, or reverses most chronic illness.

The type of nutrition, 70–80 percent vegetables and fruit, 20 percent or so of meat products is critical and leads to great health. A high-sugar and nonorganic-meat way of eating would lead to poor health. Three-fourths of the plate should be starchy or nonstarchy vegetables and fruit. No diet. Yes, be mindful of the type of food you eating. Eat all you want; the vitamins, minerals, and phytochemicals will turn your appetite off.

Physical fitness is number three on the wellness wheel. You can read my chapter on that for details. One base lead to better what you're circumstances, usually, you can figure out something. You can find a lot of things on the Internet. For example, I learned about twenty or so core exercises by watching videos.

The easiest way is to increase your AOL, your activities of living; the more you can do, the better it works. Computer desk, using a stand-up desk, walking during the lunch hour, and so on are great ways to improve your AOL. Remember, if you increase your calorie burn by 200 calories per day, that is twenty pounds in a year; knowing that and eating correctly makes good health habits fairly easy. You could stop, reverse, and avoid most chronic illness that way. Besides you'll feel just great. I also recommend light weight lifting, perhaps in combination with yoga, which makes it a lot easier. If you are in a wheelchair, you can do a lot of things to strengthen your arms if they're okay. I run a wheelchair tennis tournament every year, and every one of these participants looks very healthy. At home I have pictures of thirty-five of them, and I'm proud of every one of them.

Spirituality is number four on the wellness wheel. To some people it would be number one. Wellness is taught in *The Daniel Plan*, The book was written by Rick Warren and links religion, the culture of the Bible, and wellness. I've taught it that way in churches, and it's very effective. Some of us need religion to change our habits. There are a lot of quotes in the Bible that can be used for that. The Daniel Plan uses the five F's: faith, food, fitness, family, and focus. It has been proven in my experience of fifty years of being a doctor that patients do better if they have faith and spirituality. That has been my experience. Incidentally, I prayed with patients periodically before surgery when their spiritual advisor was present and sometimes without. I always respected the patients' religion, not mine. I encourage the nurses to participate in this also. My next recommendation for you is to treat wellness as a way of life. Involve friends, family, your workplace, and everyone around you. It can be electric and spread to other people. You can help them, and they can encourage you. That way at least to view I looking at what you eating and whether you exercising or not living up to what you say. Look at it from a social, mental, work, and ethical point of view. Some would even say to have some responsibility for the body that God gave you.

When does our education as a human begin? Some would say at birth. Actually, it starts before conception. What the parents put in their fingers, what they eat, what they are exposed to in the environment, and how they use their feet affects their genetic expression. The field of epigenetics, which has been written about for only about fifteen years, tells us that 90 percent of our genes are modifiable by the abovementioned activities. So that can be good or bad news depending on what you're doing.

Number seven on the wellness wheel is integrating the mind-body-spirit connection. Dr. Candace Pert, in a famous book, *Molecules of Emotion*, published in 1972, proved how through hormones, neurotransmitters, and neuropeptides we can speak to arrive body. She discovered the opiate receptors. That's the first time we found out how we speak to our body cells.

Our seventy trillion body cells have receptors on them, and she was the first to describe them. She discovered the opiate receptor sites Psychiatrists have noted that 50 percent of the patients going to their doctor actually have mild, moderate, or severe depression, but the symptoms that decorated as something else—headaches, irritable bowel, skin rashes, and so on.

What this says is that 50 percent of the people are misdiagnosed and have a lot of procedures done to them when it is actually depression that is the problem. Frankly, they are misdiagnosed. That is because they don't understand and are not taught about the mind-body connection. It's "pill for the ill," so you must be aware of this. You could be sent on a road of injections, pills, and maybe even some unnecessary surgery. Depression may be the real problem. As already mentioned, very few providers understand the mind-body connection. Read *Molecules of Emotion*, by Candace Pert, and *Welcome to your Mind Body*, by Dr. Rudy Kachmann.

Lastly, it goes without saying we need to have our HRA, health risk assessment, and blood testing done by a provider, and not just every few years. I say yearly starting at birth. Then we could actually practice preventative medicine. We can avoid prediabetes, diabetes, and their secondary chronic diseases with very serious complications, including sudden death.

So HRA and blood testing is critical. Read Dr. Mark Hyman's *How to Speak to Your Doctor* free on the Internet. You can copy it, and it's just great and very helpful.

AOL: Activity of Living

like to use the acronym AOL—activities of living—for the energy burn we undergo pursuing our daily life. I consider it separate from our BMR, which is the energy used up by the lungs, heart, files, brain, and muscles at rest, doing nothing.

Dr. John Levine from the Mayo Clinic assembled a team of one hundred scientists and studied the activities of living, separate from exercise. They did great studies. His team and the Mayo Clinic called it NEAT, nonexercise activity thermogenesis. They legally own the name. They published their findings, and Dr. John Levine wrote a great book about it called *Move a Little, Lose a Lot*. He lectured all over the world and was on TV many times going back at least a decade.

I include regular exercise programs inside AOL. The reason is that researchers have found only 3.5 to 5 percent of people exercise regularly. They follow them. I think that simplifies advising people what to do.

I am surprised that in spite of Dr. John Levine's work in the Mayo Clinic behind him that our obesity rate is actually increasing. Personally, I think the Mayo Clinic's advice on diabetes prevention has been too soft. I think using sitting disease, explaining it, and then using proper nutrition and increasing your AOL is a fairly easy way to improve your health and should be pushed by major healthcare providers. Let's face it: we're facing an epidemic.

Eat a nutrient-dense diet and increase your AOL to prevent, stop, and reverse type 2 diabetes 90 percent of the time in about thirty to sixty days, a high percentage actually in thirty days. Some even can get rid of a lot of their medicines in a few weeks, saving themselves a lot of money and chronic illnesses in the future.

I encourage you to read *Goodbye Diabetes*, by Dr. Youngberg; *The 30-Day Miracle*, by Franklin House; *End of Diabetes*, by Dr. Joel Fuhrman; and *Secret of the None Diet* and *Reversing Diabetes*, by Dr. Rudy Kachmann. Also, visit Kachmannhealth.com for 120 free one-hour YouTube lectures.

Dr. Levine noted that Dr. Claude Bouchard in 1990 published some studies of twelve sets of twins, that he fed a thousand extra calories for three months. They did not exercise and were in a dormitory. The average weight gain was eighteen pounds—but the range was from nine to thirty pounds. So Dr. Levine thought there were NEAT genes.

So he ran his own study. He assembled a team of a hundred scientists. For two months and the item was food was measured, they had five cooks. They also fed a thousand extra calories. Fifteen people were used. Some gained nothing; one of them gained fourteen pounds. They figured that the BMR could not have changed that much.

To solve the mystery, they designed NEAT underwear to pick up every vibration occurring in the body. The technology was inspired by NASA. They used micro sensors. Sitting, standing, walking, climbing, and so on were studied. Instruments were used to translate the action took calorie burn.

They determined that if an overweight person did the same AOL or NEAT as a lean person, he or she could burn an extra 350 calories, which translated into thirty-five pounds in a year. What's interesting is that it would take one hour of extremely vigorous gym activity a day to do the same. And remember, only 3.5 percent of people exercise regularly, and they do so at a fairly normal pace, not extreme exercise. So they and I conclude it's a lot easier to figure out how to increase your AOL or NEAT. Turn the switch on, and increase your AOL. A solid combination of food selection and increasing your AOL, not just total calories, will be a huge step in the right direction.

Remember, calories in is not calories out. A high vegetable-and-fruit way of eating will eliminate 30–50 percent of calories because the foods are water dense and high fiber, and a high rate of metabolism will remove a lot of the calories.

Make a list of your AOL activities, keep it on the wall in the office or at home, use your imagination, and think of new ways to do it. Especially at work in your increase your free time at home, maybe even increasing your ability to increase your AOL there.

Encourage your employer to buy you a treadmill desk or stand-up desk. Don't sit more than twenty minutes, then move around, maybe do some squats, keep some light weights at your desk, and take a walk whenever you can. Take a walk on your lunch hour if you can. Use the stairs. Find a friend to walk with. Make AOL or NEAT the office culture.

List of AOL activities:

- Use a stand-up desk
- Use a treadmill with a computer
- Use the stairs
- Keep light weights by your desk
- Do some lunges and squats at your desk
- Hold on and stand on one leg in a lunge for squat position
- Stand up and dance when cooking
- Take a daily thirty-minute walk
- Get a dog
- Play a fun sport
- Join a workout place if you can
- Do yoga, tai chi—develop a routine
- Correctly use some light weights
- Count the number of hours that you are sitting
- Stand up when the phone rings
- Find a friend that's doing the same thing
- Visualize the result you're looking for daily
- Remember that a habit takes on average twenty-one days to become permanent
- Start counting your steps, record the number of times you stand up – set a goal

CHILDREN AND SITTING DISEASE

Unfortunately, our children have a major problem with sitting disease. It has been found that teenagers and even younger children are on the Internet on average about nine hours a day. They're on Facebook, Twitter, Snapchat, social media, iPhones, and whatever the latest communicative technology might be. I just read the story of a popular teenager in a California high school that eventually committed suicide. The best they could figure he was up night after night with technology and rarely slept. He was very popular and lived with a good family, and they could not come up with any other reason.

I personally surveyed a hundred teenagers and asked them to estimate the percentage of time they spent using technology that they were sitting or lying down. The average answer was 80–90 percent of the time. Teenagers clearly have sitting disease.

No wonder we're looking at an increase in children who are overweight, even obese, with the usual complications at a very young age. They'll have heart disease, diabetes, metabolic diseases, and increased rates of cancer at a very young age, sometimes in their forties, thirties, and even twenties. Type 2 diabetes, as you know, has been increasing yearly. Premature deaths, heart attacks, strokes, diabetes, high blood pressure, deep vein thrombosis, and certain cancers are increasing yearly in younger children and young adults. The majority of those illnesses are preventable.

Some parents are tracking their children by putting pedometers on them to get some idea of how many steps they are taking. This is a great idea. One of my grandchildren now is taking at least ten thousand steps a day. Incidentally, 20 steps are equal to 1 calorie burned.

Researchers found that children between the ages of nine and eleven who spend 75 percent of their time engaged in sedentary actions such as watching TV or using technology are more likely to exhibit poor motor coordination than more active children in the same age range.

Several schools now offer stand-up desks or just. Students can stand up during a class and so on. This needs to happen throughout the country. School boards need to have a look at this and make it a policy in their districts. Most chronic illnesses and habits begin at a young age. Monica Wendell, director of the Center of Community Health at Texas A&M, has put stand-up desks in four first-grade classrooms. She's found it actually improved attention on task behavior, including increased alertness and classroom engagement.

The standing revolution has even begun to spread in universities. Some of the faculty at Ohio State have brought in standing desks and recommend them for companies they deal with. In addition, they have mobilized a stand-up employer campaign. This is all wonderful work, all designed to unseat their deskbound employees. They are recommending standing at meetings or while talking on the phone, which has now become a normal action at some of them floras they deal with.

A recent large study reported that children across the globe sit for 8.5 hours every day. A very similar result to a you a study, which revealed nine hours.

Another study found that activity levels among children in the U.S. dropped precipitously after age eight and continued to fall through adolescence, with people trading movement for sitting. The study concluded this decline was most pronounced among girls.

They then studied the vascular system of nine- to twelve-year-olds with ultrasounds and blood pressure cuffs. One-half of the girls sat for three hours in a laboratory with iPads, watched movies, and so on. The other girls also sat for three hours but exercised on a bike for at least ten minutes each hour. The girls sitting without exercise had a profound decrease in vascular function. Vascular dilatation fell by as much as 33 percent.

Promoting low-level activity and reducing sitting time throughout the school day may be the key to improving the health of our children. Some schools even have stationary bikes with desks attached to them. What a great idea. Most classroom learning can be done while standing, pedaling, and so on. In the state of the month the encouraging children to exercise an additional thirty minutes a day besides gym activity. The clearly by integrating physical activity into the classroom setting up. This is happening in elementary and middle schools. There are good scientific studies to support that. There have not been many studies done for teenagers.

We need to give educators the tools to encourage children to increase their movement and develop a lifestyle accordingly. This could be a way of educating the whole country on good health habits and disease prevention. This is a great opportunity for all of us because we're facing a 70–90 percent chronic illness rate. It could break the country. Teachers who allowed stand-up desks, stationary bicycles with desks, standing and stretching for the students are showing kindness and wisdom to their children.

Summary

Sitting disease is a metabolic syndrome where the enzyme LPL, in the endothelial layer of your blood vessels after sixty to ninety minutes of inactivity turns off about 50%. This enzyme controls triglyceride and glucose metabolism throughout your three hundred thousand miles of capillaries. Do you have sitting disease? Count up the hours you're driving, watching TV, sitting at work, and so on. Study for a few days your activity level, and average out your sitting time. Then do the same for your children. I read and write a lot at Starbucks, and that certainly is sitting. Then again, I work out two hours a day because I have more time now, as I'm semiretired.

Workers who manage people generally sit about 70 percent of the day. Certainly, some are lucky and are walking around the office or factory all day long. Some sit 90 percent of the time. Those of you working at a factory and walking all day may not think you're lucky, but I think you can be very fortunate as it can lead to great health. Let's face it: if you're healthy, you're worth at least $1 million. You can be worth $1 billion, but if you are not healthy, you actually have very little. I know a number of very rich executives; the majority of them are in poor health from bad habits. They are very intelligent but blind to their own reality.

We are structured to move. If you're not moving, your body goes to sleep. This includes your enzymes and the rest of your metabolic activity. This is not how we were designed to be.

As already mentioned many times, most chronic diseases, including dementia, heart attacks, strokes, diabetes, cancer, and bowel and autoimmune diseases, are a result of poor diet and lack of exercise. Even exercising one day a week at a workout center will not make much difference if you sit eight to ten hours a day and eat a poor-nutrient diet.

I recommend that you read that chapter on your total daily calorie burn a number of times. I really want you to understand that because that's the easiest way to great health. Frankly, if you increase your AOL and pay attention to the type of food you eat—70–80 percent nutrient-dense foods such as vegetables and fruits and 20 percent organic meats—you will be very healthy. You will have a normal weight, avoid most chronic illnesses, and live to be a hundred. No canes, no wheelchairs, and no nursing homes. Besides, you'll have a great memory that is as good as you can possibly have at that age. Frankly, it's not that difficult.

Good luck,

Dr. Wellness (Rudy Kachmann, MD)

About the Author

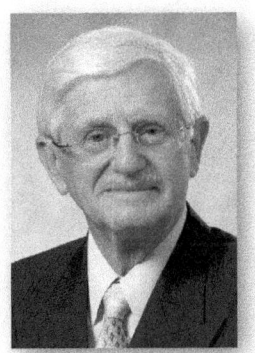

Rudy Kachmann, MD, is a renowned medical expert, author, lecturer, keynote speaker, neurosurgeon, television host, and Kachmann Mind Body Institute medical director. His forty-two years of experience practicing neurology and neurosurgery include over ten thousand brain and spine operations and more than forty thousand treated patients.

Presently, he is the medical director of wellness for Lutheran Health Network and gives roughly forty mind body health lectures per year. Dr. Kachmann also has two weekly television shows focusing on wellness.